ANTI-OPPRESSIVE PRACTICE

This

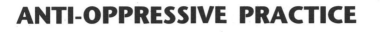

ANTI-OPPRESSIVE PRACTICE

Social care and the law

JANE DALRYMPLE AND
BEVERLEY BURKE

Open University Press
Maidenhead • Philadelphia

Open University Press
McGraw-Hill House
Shoppenhangers Road
Maidenhead
Berkshire
England
SL6 2QL

email: enquiries@openup.co.uk
world wide web: www.openup.co.uk

and
325 Chestnut Street
Philadelphia, PA 19106, USA

First Published 1995
Reprinted 1996 (twice), 1997, 1998, 1999 (twice), 2000, 2001, 2003

A catalogue record of this book is available from the British Library

ISBN 0 335 19193 2 (pb)

Library of Congress Cataloging-in-Publication Data

Dalrymple, Jane, 1951–
    Anti-oppressive practice : social care and the law / by Jane Dalrymple and Beverley Burke.
        p. cm.
    Includes bibliographical references and index.
    ISBN 0–335–19193–2
    1. Social service—Great Britain.   2. Public welfare—Law and legislation—Great Britain.   I. Burke, Beverley, 1957–   .
II. Title.
HV245.D24   1995   94–26582
361.941—dc20   CIP

Typeset by Graphicraft Limited, Hong Kong
Printed by Bell & Bain Ltd., Glasgow

Dedicated to June Henfrey and Margaret Simey

For the effect of her being on those around her was incalcu-
lably diffusive; for the growing good of the world is partly
dependent on unhistoric acts; and that things are not so ill
with you and me as they might have been, is half owing to the
number who lived faithfully a hidden life, and rest in unvisited
tombs.

George Eliot: *Middlemarch*

CONTENTS

LIST OF STATUTES

Access to Personal Files Act 1987
Adoption Act 1984
Children Act 1989
Child Support Act 1991
Chronically Sick and Disabled Persons Act 1970
Criminal Justice Act 1991
Disabled Persons Act 1986
Education Act 1985
Education Act 1993
Housing Act 1985
Local Government Act 1988
Mental Health Act 1983
Mental Health Act 1989
National Assistance Act 1948
National Health Service Act 1977
National Health Service and Community Care Act 1990
Race Relations Act 1976

LIST OF CASES

FOREWORD

Almost three decades since the first piece of equal opportunities legislation was enacted, the authors of this treatise on anti-discrimination and anti-oppressive practices in social care attempt to rationalize the journey so far and proffer suggestions.

Between the Scylla of autonomy of law and the Charybdis of law of economics and therefore the will of the dominant group in society, they steer a *via media*: that law is relatively autonomous and, indeed, could be used to promote good social work practice. I find this strategy of argumentation (even though it is not beyond the reach of criticism) intellectually stimulating. In pursuit of this strategy, the concept of empowerment and the various aspects of social care practice, such as partnership, assessment, planning, user involvement and evaluation, are contextualized, taking cognizance of relevant case studies, case law and statutes.

It must be stressed, however, that this is not a treatise on the law relating to anti-discrimination and anti-oppressive practices but a presentation of concepts, theories, case studies, case law, statutes and assignments that aims to amplify the lessons of social care practice.

Solomon E. Salako, LL M (London), M.Phil (London), ACIS, Barrister
Senior Lecturer in Law, Liverpool John Moores University

PREFACE

The initial inspiration for this book sprang from a request by Guy Mitchell to write an article for *Panel News*. It was entitled 'Implementing race and culture issues using the Children Act 1989'. We were concerned in writing the article to encourage our readers to seize the opportunities presented by that Act to improve the situation for black young people and their families. In the writing of that article we reflected on our own practice, which consequently stimulated debate with friends, colleagues and students with whom we were working at the time. It was through these debates that we changed our own perceptions of the law and began to realize that by using it constructively it is possible to enable people to make changes in their lives. This is not to deny the fact that some of the legislation must be challenged, or is of itself oppressive and can deny people their liberty. Such is the contradictory nature of the legislation. We see this book as a guide through the contradictions and our contribution to the process of change.

Jane Dalrymple initially undertook her social work training at the Josephine Butler College in Liverpool and has practised as a social worker since. More recently she has worked for a charity which seeks to challenge oppressive practice concerning children and young people. Beverley Burke was formerly a social worker, for many years in a local authority intake team, and now lectures in social work at the Josephine Butler House, Liverpool John Moores University. Josephine Butler is one of the threads that link our lives. Through our discussions we have discovered that the link of Josephine Butler reminded us of the history of women's struggle and our own contribution to the struggle against oppression. This book is dedicated to two women whose own 'sense of outrage' and struggle against oppression has inspired us. We were both fortunate to know June Henfrey and have been able to share some thoughts about this book with Margaret Simey. We have been inspired by the lives and work of both women.

We are also indebted to family, friends and colleagues who have provided us with emotional support and space, and encouraged us to complete the work. Special thanks are due to all those who have read different chapters of the book and those who have discussed ideas with us. Particular thanks are due to Chris Hardwick and Brian Scott, who cast their critical literary eyes over our work, and Solomon Salako for his encouragement. The book would not be complete without the poetic contributions of Chrissie Elms Bennett and Chris Kwaku Kyem and we appreciate their willingness to share with us their experiences. Finally we have to thank Jo Campling, who saw the potential and encouraged us to write.

NOTES ON TERMINOLOGY

We provide the following definitions as an aid to the terms we use in the text. The very act of defining brings with it a set of problems. But it is important that we attempt to come to some common understanding as this aids communication. The following are not exhaustive definitions but ones we have used to guide our thinking.

Adultism

We use the term 'adultism' to mean the oppression of children and young people by adults. Adults have power over children and young people and so we feel that this more forcefully states the power differential that exists between them. The alternative word that could be used is 'ageism'. However, this is more commonly understood as a word applying to the oppression of older people: 'Ageism means unwarranted application of negative stereotypes to older people' (Fennell *et al.* 1988: 97).

Black

We follow Bandana Ahmad's (1990) terminology in use of the word 'black', which is used to describe people mainly from South Asian, African and Caribbean backgrounds and other visible minorities in Britain. We do not use the term 'black' to deny difference and diversity. The term 'black' is used in a political sense to reflect the struggles of non-white groups against the oppression they experience from white institutions. The expression of being 'black' is a source of unified strength and solidarity.

Discrimination

Discrimination is a term which is linked to the legislative framework. It has been defined as 'unfair or unequal treatment of individuals or groups; prejudicial behaviour acting against the interests of those people who characteristically tend to belong to relatively powerless groups within the social structure (women, ethnic minorities, old or disabled people, and members of the working class in general). Discrimination is therefore a matter of social formation as well as individual/group behaviour or praxis' (Thompson 1993: 31). 'Legislation against discrimination is fundamentally reformist in orientation, for it is concerned with promoting small scale changes, rather than any fundamental restructuring of power relationships or social values.' Consequently 'anti-discriminatory practice will work to a model of challenging unfairness' (Phillipson 1992: 14).

Gillick competent

A Gillick competent child or young person is one who has sufficient understanding to make decisions for himself or herself. The Children Act 1989 makes it a statutory responsibility to take into account the wishes and feelings of the child or young person concerned. This is a recognition of the decision in *Gillick* v *West Norfolk and Wisbech Area Health Authority* [1986] AC 112, where the House of Lords discussed the relationship between the parent and child and the responsibilities that arise from that relationship. Although the judgment related to consent to medical treatment the principle applies to decision making on any important matter.

The judgment indicated that there is a tapering relationship between parents and their children. Thus as children become older and more mature the parents' rights to know about their affairs, and to make decisions on their behalf, diminishes. Children therefore do not have to wait for the age of majority (18) to be able to decide matters for themselves – that informed choice can be made at an earlier age.

A number of cases have subsequently caused confusion in respect of the law concerning the concept of informed consent. However, the term 'Gillick competent' has remained and embodies a child's or young person's right to growing self-determination (Brayne and Martin 1990).

Oppression

The word oppress comes from the Latin *opprimere*, which means to press on, or to press against. It has been defined as 'Inhuman or degrading treatment of individuals or groups; hardship and injustice brought about by the dominance of one group over another; the negative and demeaning exercise of power. Oppression often involves disregarding the rights of an individual or group and is thus the denial of citizenship' (Thompson 1993: 31). Anti-oppressive practice 'works with a model of empowerment and liberation and requires a fundamental rethinking of values, institutions and relationships' (Phillipson 1992: 15).

Social care

'This term is used to describe the activities and processes undertaken by all sectors or agencies (statutory, voluntary and independent) which seek to enable individuals, families and groups who are disadvantaged or deprived in some way to achieve a higher, self-determined level of functioning and quality of life. It is about the planned meeting of clients' needs. It concerns the physical, intellectual, emotional, cultural and social aspects of the client's development and well-being. It involves mutual trust and respect; it involves a sense of purpose and change; it recognises the interaction between people and their environments' (Mallinson 1988: 1). We use the term 'social care' to cover all the activities of caring that are undertaken by health and welfare workers and informal carers.

INTRODUCTION

The law is an instrument and not an end in itself. If you learn
how to use the law you can do something with it.
> (Margaret Simey in an interview with the authors,
> November 1993)

Asked what it was that gave her the strength to continue her work, Josephine
Butler replied that it was 'the awful abundance of compassion which makes
me fierce'. Josephine Butler was born in 1828. Committed to fighting injustice and oppression, she spent the greater part of her life campaigning against
legislation regulating prostitution. It has been said that if

> Josephine Butler were alive today, she would still be campaigning against
> sexual exploitation. She would be arguing with passion against pornog-
> raphy. She would be out amongst the drug addicts, the AIDS-sufferers,
> the prostitutes of both sexes, loving them and caring for them. But at
> the same time she would be ruthless in her exposure of those who
> exploited and trapped them.
>
> (*Church Times*, 26 December 1986)

Biographers have stated that Josephine was not a born fighter, neither stimulated by public action nor thriving on confrontation. She was not considered
a natural candidate to lead a public cause or to be a social worker.

Compassion is not perhaps a word that many would use to describe their
motivation for working in health and social care practice. However, compassion can be described as 'sharing', and if you share the distress of people
then you cannot walk away (Simey 1993). Margaret Simey has spent her life
dedicated to the people of Merseyside. Her work has been based in the
Granby area of Merseyside, where she has spoken out boldly but wisely
against what she has seen as injustice and oppression. In September 1993,

talking to students at Josephine Butler House, Liverpool John Moores University, she described Josephine's 'blistering sense of outrage' not only as the quality which made her 'fierce' but also as the quality which has been lost in much social care practice. 'Compassion fatigue' is defined as 'indifference to human suffering as a result of over exposure to charitable appeals' (*Reader's Digest Oxford Complete Wordfinder*). Social care practice reflects society and so, for some, the sense of outrage has been replaced by indifference. This is one of the reasons why we have actively sought to use the law to inform a practice that is anti-oppressive rather than something apart. We do not need to be 'born fighters'. However, we do need a commitment to anti-oppressive practice – a fierceness born from both compassion and a sense of outrage, not 'compassion fatigue'.

Our practice is grounded in the law, but there is a gap between practice and theory. The law should not be seen as something apart from what we do but as something which should be used to *inform* practice. We will consider the positive elements of the law and try to work on those which are hidden, building on them rather than seeing the law as totally constraining. This will be achieved by consideration of some of the principles that underpin the legislation which impinges on health and welfare practice. We are not saying that the law is perfect or that some of the ideologies underpinning the law cannot or should not be challenged. What we are saying is that work in the social care field is dominated by the law, so we should seek to use it to inform a practice that is anti-oppressive.

The book is written in three parts. The first part sets the terms of the debate. In Chapter 1 we begin to unpack the concepts of power and oppression which underpin anti-oppressive practice in order to develop a theory that informs our practice. Chapter 2 goes on to look at why we have chosen to use the vehicle of the law to promote anti-oppressive practice. We suggest that health and social care practitioners and carers either work within the constraints of the law and accept the dominant ideology underpinning legislation, or use the law to challenge the inequalities present in society, which can be further perpetuated through legislation. The chapter considers the contradictions and dilemmas that are present in legislation and develops an argument for using it as a radical tool.

By the end of Part I you should have an understanding of the theories and ideologies informing anti-oppressive practice and legislation. This provides the backdrop for Part II, where we go on to look at some of the elements we consider important in a model for anti-oppressive practice. Chapter 3 begins this process by discussing the value base of the law. It is important to be aware of the values which inform legislation in order to negotiate successfully its contradictory elements. For us the exploration of one's personal values is a starting point for anti-oppressive practice and we use our own experience to develop this. We hope, therefore, that those involved in the delivery of social care services can begin their own self-exploration as a part of the process of understanding anti-oppressive practice.

Having considered the importance of a firm value base, we then go on in Chapter 4 to look at empowerment, a vital element of anti-oppressive practice. It is necessary to think about what exactly this means to both workers and service users. Partnership encompasses the power relationships that exist between families, professional workers, carers and the state. Chapter 5 therefore considers partnership, and links to the discussions about empowerment in the previous chapter. We look at how the power relationships that exist within partnerships can be used to ensure that the rights of everyone involved are upheld. Partnership includes, among other things, the joint planning of services to ensure not only that users have choice but that intervention can be kept to a minimum. We consider minimal intervention in practice in Chapter 6 and conclude Part II by drawing these elements together into a model of anti-oppressive practice.

If intervention is to be kept to a minimum then practitioners and carers need to develop skills in assessment and planning, in order to make decisions with service users about what is in their best interests. Part III draws on the theory and principles presented in Parts I and II to reframe practice in relation to legislation. In the next three chapters we therefore consider practice in relation to preventive work, assessment and planning, addressing the importance of user involvement throughout the process.

If we are committed to anti-oppressive practice then it is vital that we continually question the work in which we are engaged. This is particularly important if users and carers are to be provided with the best possible service. By evaluating our work we take account of the needs of service users, and challenge and develop our practice wisdom. We have striven in writing this book to ensure that it is not just a theoretical exposition. Essentially it is practice based and looks at the reality of anti-oppressive practice.

At this point we need to note the distinction between anti-oppressive and anti-discriminatory practice. It is important to make this distinction, as all too often the terms are used interchangeably, without thought being given to the impact of both terms. For us anti-oppressive practice is about minimizing the power differences in society. Such practice 'works with a model of empowerment and liberation and requires a fundamental rethinking of values, institutions and relationships' (Phillipson 1992: 15). Legislation which deals with issues of discrimination – such as the Race Relations or the Sex Discrimination Acts – is *specific* and aimed at addressing unfair treatment faced, for example, by black people or women. Anti-discriminatory practice uses particular legislation to *challenge* the discrimination faced by some groups of people.

Anti-discriminatory and anti-oppressive practice can complement each other. We do not deny the usefulness of anti-discriminatory practice but we feel that it is limiting in its potential to challenge power differentials. It is important for us to develop a practice which ultimately addresses structural inequalities.

By way of illustration of this point consider the following scenario. A white worker is working with a black family. Issues arise which the white worker feels unable to address. The worker therefore uses legislation to ensure that a black worker is allocated to the case. Working from an *anti-discriminatory* perspective, the worker quite rightly uses the means available to address the problem. A worker using an *anti-oppressive* perspective would also use the legislation to ensure that the needs of the family were being met. He or she would say, however, that it is not enough just to have a black worker allocated. There are other, wider issues that need to be considered which go beyond the specific situation. There are implications for future practice. For example, these are some of the issues that should be addressed:

- Why was a white worker allocated in the first place?
- How many black workers does the agency employ?
- What training have the workers had?
- It is important that white workers do not abdicate their responsibilities.
- There is a need for black and white workers to work in partnership.
- There is a need to acknowledge the strengths and expertise of individual workers.

While we are using the law as an empowering tool we are aware of the contradictions that exist. For example, there is legislation which discriminates *against* certain groups of people, such as gays, lesbians or travellers. Immigration legislation is used to control and regulate the lives of certain groups of people. Campaigns for anti-discriminatory legislation by people with disabilities continue to be ignored. We acknowledge all these anomalies. However, the focus of this book is to consider how a range of legislation can be used to empower people and combat their oppression.

There is a wealth of legislation available to health and welfare practitioners and carers. We have not attempted to cover all available legislation and it will be seen that we have made scant reference to benefits or housing legislation, for example. Both of these have an impact on health and social care practice, often in conjunction with other pieces of legislation. For instance, while looking at the Children Act in relation to the needs of homeless young people we could have discussed the necessity for young people to be given an adequate income to enable them to maintain their accommodation. This would have led us to an examination of the inadequacy of the benefits legislation and the need for changes to be made. It is important to be aware of the interconnections between pieces of legislation which can often contradict and be confusing. However, it is beyond the scope of this book to complete a total analysis of all legislation that pertains to social care practice.

We believe that it is not possible to explore the concepts of oppression and anti-oppressive practice without sharing our experiences and expertise as women and as social work practitioners. The book reflects this, in that issues of race and gender feature more than, say, ageism and disabilism. And we have also used legislation with which we are most familiar, such as the National Health Service and Community Care Act 1990 and the Children Act 1989, to provide pointers to using the law to promote anti-oppressive practice. The essence of this book, however, is encapsulated in the words of Margaret Simey at the beginning of this introduction, and we hope that, having read it, you will be able to use the law as a positive force for change.

Part I UNPACKING CONCEPTS:

SETTING THE TERMS

OF THE DEBATE

1   SOME ESSENTIAL

ELEMENTS OF

ANTI-OPPRESSIVE THEORY

> The focus of revolutionary change is never merely the oppressive
> situations which we seek to escape, but that piece of the
> oppressor which is planted deep within each of us, and which
> knows only the oppressors' tactics, the oppressors' relationships.
> (Lorde 1984: 123)

Empowerment

Why do they speak to me this way?
What happened to my right to have my say?
Why do they speak to me this way?
What happened to my right to protection?
Why do they reject and push me away?
What happened to my opinion and viewpoints?
Why do they assess me this way?
What happened to my freedom I must say?
Why do they label me this way?
What happened to my right to the things I do?
Why do they take everything from me this way?
What happened to my possessions? feelings? emotions?
Why do they act this way?
What happened to my rights? –
They took them away.
What I need is more power.
Please let us stand together,
because I don't want to fight you.

(Chrissie Elms Bennett 1994)

Chrissie's poem is written from her experiences as a young person in residential care. It is an account of her feelings of powerlessness. We will all have

experienced powerlessness at some time in our lives: perhaps as children we felt powerless when told off by an adult; perhaps as adults we have felt powerless because we have been unemployed, or, if in work, we have been told to do something by managers that we feel unhappy about. In such situations we experience a whole range of emotions, and it is these feelings of powerlessness that provide the starting point for an understanding of oppression and power.

For us, the starting point is our experience of being women in a society that does not value the many contributions that women have made and are making. Not all women are viewed as equal. Black women are treated differently from white women, lesbian women are treated differently from heterosexual women, disabled women are viewed differently from able-bodied women, older women are viewed differently from younger women. The society that we live in is characterized by 'difference' but these differences are not always seen positively. Differences are used to *exclude* rather than include. This is because relationships within society are the result of the exercise of power on individual, interpersonal and institutional levels.

While writing, we have explored the various points of difference that exist between us. We have been able to name and understand our oppression based on 'race', gender and class. We have also been enabled to develop a fuller and richer understanding of who we are and what we mean to each other. It is not easy to explore points of divergence, for each display of our personal vulnerabilities in turn is a loss if we are honest of some personal power – our credibility. In order to engage in discussions around power and oppression one has to have personal strength and be committed to change. Changing one's behaviour – once it has been identified as being oppressive – is about being open to the views of others and being committed to the process of change.

This chapter reflects our individual experiences of *being*. For one of us it is the experience of being black, female and heterosexual, with a working-class background but located in a middle-class occupation and enjoying a lifestyle that reflects the benefits conferred by that position. For the other it is the experience of being white, heterosexual, female and middle class. By telling our own stories to each other we have engaged in the first step 'in freeing oneself from oppression' (Kolb-Morris 1993: 100). By locating ourselves through the process of self-definition we show our commitment to changing actively the world in which we live.

In our exploration of the issues of oppression and, therefore, our understanding of power we draw heavily on literature written by women, particularly black women. Black women have played a specific role in documenting their experiences of oppression: 'in the struggle for racial justice this contribution has been underplayed in the past but presents rich possibilities' (Henfrey 1988: 192). We open up these possibilities by reflecting and focusing upon our experiences of being women as well as the experiences of other women. We make no apology for this bias, for we believe that the ideas and issues that we explore can be extended to other oppressed groups and that women have made a unique contribution to the understanding of oppression.

If work with people who have limited power or who are marginalized is to be effective then it should link the personal realities of people's lives to the structural context in which they exist. By incorporating the concepts of power and oppression within a theoretical framework, it is possible within our work to build on the strengths, rather than the deficiencies, of individuals. The law is a powerful resource which can be used to develop our practice – it is important to engage with it, transform it and use it in a creative and meaningful way. If the potential of the legislation is to be realized then we need to have a clear understanding of it.

This book is about anti-oppressive practice. In this chapter, through an analysis of what is meant by *power* and *oppression*, we lay the foundations of a *theory* which considers the ideas and assumptions about the relationships we have with each other.

Why is it important to have theories for practice?

In order to practise effectively we need to have a view about what we are doing. If we are going to swim against the tide we have to be strong enough to survive. What gives us our strength as anti-oppressive practitioners is our view of the world. This view guides our actions. As Malcolm Payne (1991: 1) says in relation to social work practice, 'to take part in social work you need a view about what you are doing – an interim view perhaps, but something which guides the actions you take'. Payne (1991: 52) goes on to suggest that theory offers:

- *models* describing what happens during practice in a general way, applying to a wide range of situations, and in a structured way, so that they extract certain principles and patterns of activity which give the practice consistency;
- *approaches to* or *perspectives on* a complex human activity which allow participants to order their minds sufficiently to be able to manage themselves while participating;
- *explanations* which account for why an action results in particular consequences, and circumstances in which it does so;
- *prescriptions* for actions so that workers know what to do when faced with particular circumstances;
- *accountability* to managers, politicians, clients and public by describing acceptable practice sufficiently to enable social work activities to be checked to see that they are appropriate;
- *justifications* for the use of the models and explanations of practice.

Many practitioners find it difficult to link theory and practice or to acknowledge the importance of any theoretical framework. However, it is important to make the connections between the ideas that inform our practice and the practice itself. Smid and van Krieken (1984) address the dilemmas experienced by practitioners in relating theory to practice, in order to enable practitioners to recognize that theorizing goes on all the time in various ways and at different levels. They developed a typology of three levels of theorizing which we find helpful in thinking through how theory affects our practice.

Materialist social theory is the first level, and provides a general picture of how society is organized. This includes consensus or conflict explanations of society. In our development of anti-oppressive theory you will find that we personally subscribe to a conflict explanation of society. For example, if we look at aspects of funding for small voluntary organizations, what we find is that groups are put in competition with each other as they attempt to access what limited resources there are. Chorcora *et al.* (1994: 66) reflect the conflict explanations of such a situation when they state that

> there is now a belief among many that the continual need to compete for funding is just a strategy of those in powerful positions to keep the poor busy preparing their proposals, diluting their strength and motivation to band together in opposition to the faceless controllers of resources.

The second level is *strategic practice theory*, which confronts questions about how to do things. For us this may be identified, for example, in work in partnership with users, using tools such as written agreements. It is important not to divorce this level from the materialist level of theorizing. For example, when we consider the use of written agreements in Chapter 10 we have to take account of the context in which we are practising. Or, if we are considering group work as a method of working, it is important to acknowledge that it is not only an enabling process but also a political position, whose goal is the changing of existing power relations (Chorcora *et al.* 1994).

The third level is about *working concepts*, which are all the ideas and experiences which affect our practice. For example, we both continually use our own experiences as women, being black, working in organizations that are primarily managed by men, to develop our theoretical perspectives of the world in which we live. Our experiences of powerlessness in these situations enable us to reflect on the nature of power in society. This then assists us to understand the position of others who are marginalized or oppressed.

Anti-oppressive practice should respond to the reality of both users' lives and our own lives. This is at both a personal and a structural level. Therefore, the theory needs to be interactive or reflexive (Payne 1991: 22). As such it will inevitably change in response to varying historical, social, political and economic factors.

We feel that it is important for practitioners to theorize their work if it is to be effective. For us, two important elements of anti-oppressive theory are the concepts of power and oppression. Both of these are subjects in their own right and books have been written on both (Friere 1972; Lukes 1974, 1986; Solomon 1976). What we present, however, is an introduction to the theoretical concepts. In no way is this a comprehensive exposition but it aims to provide an initial framework which can be developed. This will require further reading, personal analysis and discussion with friends and colleagues for you to be able to develop a theory and practice which you can acknowledge as your own.

Reflections on theory and practice

> We have been told that poetry expresses what we feel, and theory states what we know ... we have been told that poetry has a soul and theory has a mind and that we have to choose between them.
>
> (Nancy Bereano, in Lorde 1984: 8)

But do we have to choose? The world is experienced not only through the level of ideas but also through the level of feelings. These levels we explore in more detail in Chapter 4. Poetry and theory are not mutually exclusive, but different parts that make up a richer explanation of the world that we live in. The exploration of feelings as well as an intellectual explanation of the world that we inhabit is what is important. Through this exploration we provide a way of both seeing and understanding the practice of social care, a practice that seeks to empower both those who require services and those who provide a service.

In our attempts to make sense of the world we generate explanations of *why things should be the way they are*. Theories help to focus our minds. They give us a lens through which we can observe and impose consistency. They go beyond simply defining social reality to attempting to explain that reality. Theories provide 'workable definitions' of the world about us (Howe 1987: 10). They reflect the social, political and economic conditions of society. It is important to acknowledge this fact, for some ideas about the world can be given prominence and thus universally accepted, or suppressed and thus denied. Theories essentially reflect the power relationships that exist between us all.

As anti-oppressive practitioners and carers it is essential that we recognize the importance of bringing a clear perspective to the work that we do. This perspective can be defined as 'the totality of a worker's political standpoints, experiences, theoretical knowledge, their [sic] self image, experience of their training and practice, their guidelines for action – in short their practice ideologies' (Smid and van Krieken 1984: 16; quoted in Rees 1991: 74). Theories embody a set of ideas that inform our interactions with others.

Guidelines for action reflect the lived experiences of individuals. These experiences may well be born out of oppression as well as reflect domination. The experiences of individuals and groups provide only partial explanations of social reality. No one group or individual possesses 'the theory or methodology that allows it to discover the absolute "truth" ' (Hill-Collins 1990: 234) about other people's experiences. What is required is an organizing framework that allows different perspectives on the *truth* to be held.

If theories are about explanations of reality how do we go about choosing the ones that reflect most 'truth'? It is important that our selection is based on an understanding that our ideas are not neutral – they are born out of the relationship that we have with the social world. Through the process of discussion and exploration, individuals or groups are provided with the space to state their desires and in turn are listened to. From the consideration of all views a fuller understanding of reality is obtained. 'The truth about any subject only comes when all sides of the story are put together, and all their different meanings make one new one' (Alice Walker 1983; quoted in Hill-Collins 1990: 37).

This holistic perspective, brought about by the process of dialogue and the making of links, can only be obtained after the existing power differentials between groups and within groups have been addressed. Otherwise the dominant ideology will continue unchanged, denying access to alternative explanations. In our consideration of theory we have attempted to incorporate the principles of anti-oppressive practice. We do not see theory as static, just as anti-oppressive practice cannot be static. It involves us learning about ourselves, developing and moving on. For us the holistic view of human action which informs the writings of black women has shaped and informed our own female perspective of the world that we are part of. This has deepened our understanding of anti-oppressive practice and the process of empowerment.

The dual perspective

Our view of society is informed by a belief that as individuals we are connected to social structures by the thread of our lived experiences. That view is shaped by the way the society is organized. For example, our experiences as *consumers* or *providers* of health and welfare services are determined by the very way these resources are organized and distributed.

Change can only be effective if the links between the subjective experiences of people and the objective social conditions are made visible. Individuals who make the connections between their personal condition and the society in which they exist begin to make changes within themselves, within their families and community and wider social structures. Individuals who become aware of the connection between their personal condition and the society in which they exist have the means to evaluate their position critically. Through the process of self-discovery we are able to name our oppression but equally we can begin to address the causes of our oppression. Many marginalized and oppressed groups, through personal and collective struggle, have challenged oppressive practices and structures. Change is the process of social and individual interaction. To gain a better understanding of this it is important to have a view of individuals which can encompass this dual notion.

Dolores C. Norton (1978) provides a framework from which we can make sense of the complex relationships that exist between the individual and social structures. She calls this framework the dual perspective and defines it as:

> the conscious and systematic process of perceiving, understanding and comparing simultaneously the values and attitudes and behaviour of

larger societal systems with those of the client's immediate family and community system.

(Norton 1978: 3)

This idea holds that every individual is part of two systems:

1 The societal system that functions within the norms and values of the dominant groups within society.
2 The smaller system that functions in a person's immediate environment. This latter system could be the cultural system.

When the two systems do not agree concerning norms, values, expectations and ways of functioning, then difficulties arise for individuals, families and cultural groups (Johnson 1989). The process of understanding and comparison identified by Norton enables individuals to acknowledge differences as well as points of contact between the larger dominant system and the world of oppressed people. The dual perspective is a particular way of viewing the world – it is informed by a critical evaluation of the similarities and differences between the powerful and the powerless.

The perspective can inform practice with groups who have limited power and presents a way of working that is empowering. Norton uses the work of Chestang (1972) to emphasize 'the importance of an affirming attitude within the family to balance the negative effects of racial prejudice' (Kolb-Morris 1993: 102). Chestang (1972) described the black experience in terms of two interacting systems. The society at large was described as the *sustaining* system, providing an individual with status and power, this being determined by an individual's access to resources. Embedded in this is what can be called the *nurturing* system. This system provides an individual with positive images, role models and support. The nurturing within this environment of family and community provides the space for individuals to develop coping strategies. The individual is then able to develop a sense of self and thus have the resources to counteract the '*negative valuations*' (Solomon 1976; Small 1986; Ahmad 1990) placed on her or him by the dominant culture.

What do we mean by power?

The word *power* conjures up graphic imagery. It may bring about an intense emotional response. Before reading further just take a few minutes to think back to your own experiences and consider what the word power means to you.

> Those who profess to favour freedom yet deprecate agitation, are people who want crops without ploughing up the ground; They want rain without thunder and lightning. They want the ocean without the awful roar of its many waters.
>
> Power concedes nothing without demand. It never did and it never will. Find out just what any people will quietly submit to and you have found out the exact measure of injustice and wrong which will be imposed upon them, and these will continue till they are resisted with

either words or blows or both. The limits of tyrants are precise by the endurance of those whom they oppress.

(Frederick Douglas 1857; quoted in the Gypsy Survey 1993: 1)

Our understanding of the term power has been shaped by the values we hold and the ideas we have about the society we live in. It is a social concept which can be used to explore the public and private spheres of life (Barker and Roberts 1992). Barbara Solomon (1987), in her discussion about power, points out the fact that power has a number of meanings which are very much dependent on whether one deals with it from a psychological, economic, political, sociological or philosophical perspective. In her account of work with oppressed black communities in the United States of America she identifies power as 'a bridging concept which describes aspects of interpersonal relations at family, small group, organisational or community levels' (Solomon 1987: 79; quoted in Rees 1991: 36).

The usefulness of the concept of power as used by Barbara Solomon is that it can 'span the various dimensions of structural power and personal power and the inequalities and differences within different social relations. Thus structure, culture and biography can be analysed in a more integrated process' (McNay 1992: 55). Sophie Loewenstein (1976) sees power as 'the overall integrating motivational concept for all human behaviour' (as quoted by Kolb-Morris 1993: 104). She suggests that issues of power could be used to inform practice. For her the relationship between men and women, between 'races', between different social classes and between helping professionals and their clients are all variations of unequal power relations in society (Loewenstein 1976; quoted by McNay 1992: 55).

Interpretations of what is meant by power have a bearing on the practice of social care and relate to the moral issue of whose interests are being served, and who should be held accountable for the abuse of such power. Practice informed by the legitimate use of power results in an empowering practice while the 'illegitimate use of power equals professional malpractice' (Gomm 1993: 133). For example, the legitimate use of power is ensuring that service users are treated as equals in decision making processes concerning their lives, such as case conferences, ward rounds and planning meetings. Often users feel powerless in such situations, which invariably involve a large number of professional people. However, they can be empowered if those with the power are prepared to use it to ensure that the rights of the user are not infringed. On the other hand, illegitimate use of power would be to deny service users access to such forums, or to provide an illusion of involvement by only allowing them in for the latter part of a meeting. 'Empowerment and partnership must not be prizes to be given out by those with power' (Henderson 1994: 23).

No discussion of power can ignore powerlessness. Solomon (1976) identified three potential sources of powerlessness:

• the negative images which oppressed people have of themselves;
• the negative experiences that oppressed people encounter when they engage with external systems;

- systems which consistently block and deny powerless groups the opportunity to take effective action.

Powerlessness could be characterized by economic insecurity, absence of monetary support, lack of opportunity for training in critical and abstract thought, and physical and emotional stress (Sennett and Cobb 1972; Conway 1979). These aspects in turn generate *experiences* of powerlessness, such as exclusion, rejection or being treated as inferior, which lead to feelings of inadequacy, helplessness and dependency.

If we consider that people's relations are structured by power then we are less likely to stereotype, make assumptions or misinterpret other people's actions. It is when we *do* stereotype, make assumptions and misinterpret other people's actions that we start to oppress. This is eloquently described in the following excerpt:

> When I am asked if I am a 'Real Gypsy' my answer is this: I am flesh and blood, I feel pain, I feel joy, I love, I hate, cut me I bleed, I am a real human being living in today's world who happens to be a Gypsy. Not some stereotype that fits misinformed people's ideas of what a Gypsy should be.
>
> (Gypsy Survey 1993: 12)

Anti-oppressive practice, then, means recognizing power imbalances and working towards the promotion of change to redress the balance of power. In discussing student–lecturer relationships, Jeanette Henderson (1994: 19) argues, for example, that it is important not only to recognize that there is a power imbalance but also actively to work towards change – otherwise 'the educator may perpetuate inequality'. This means challenging assumptions, recognizing that we all have rights and challenging the institutional practices that oppress and so systematically disempower those with whom we work.

Oppression

> In order for the oppressed to be able to wage the struggle for their liberation they must perceive the reality of oppression, not as a closed world from which there is no exit, but as a limited situation which they can transform.
>
> (Freire 1972: 34)

It is from the experiences of people who have been marginalized, who have had their rights denied or violated, that we can understand what is meant by oppression. By listening to other people's experiences of oppression we are able to extend the parameters of what is possible (Lorde 1984). It is the *listening* that is most important, as this provides us with the information that enables us to gain a fuller understanding of the issues.

The word oppression is a value-laden term that can conjure up in our minds various disturbing images. You will probably have your own definition of what oppression means to you. Think back again to your own experiences as you consider your definition. The following extract from a poem very simply, but powerfully, demonstrates the insidious nature of oppression:

> oppression is not a choice
> or just the misfortune of the socially deprived
> no woman has escaped
> sexism like quiet rain
> constantly, softly seeping in
> until we all become saturated
> and it gently, ever so gently
> so we hardly notice
> does us terrible violence

(Aspen 1983)

This extract addresses the issue of sexism, but one could equally substitute other examples of oppression, such as racism, ageism or heterosexism. It illustrates the fact that oppression is a fact of life, based as it is on power inequality which is manifested in particular ways – in this case the differential treatment of women by men. Sexism, however, is not just an issue for women, it also affects the perpetrators – men. Sexism distorts the relationship between men and women and in the process both are violated.

There is no simple definition of oppression. It is a complex and emotive term. To seek to identify and explain it in a simple phrase is to deny its very complexity. But it is important to have a working definition of the term. Guy Mitchell (1989: 14) captures the essence of oppression as it impacts on social work practice:

> British society is saturated in oppression . . . an empowering social work practice derived from such an understanding addresses itself to the powerlessness and loss which results from the material and ideological oppression of black people by white people; working class people by middle class people, women by men; children and old people by 'adults'; disabled people by 'able' people; and gay people by 'straight' people. This social work practice recognises oppression not simply in the behaviours, values and attitudes of individuals and groups, but in the institutions, structures and common sense assumptions.

It is not only at the ideological level that oppression occurs. Political and economic structures also have a role to play. Together with ideology they function as a highly effective system of social control. In our terms, oppression can be seen 'as a state of affairs in which life chances are constructed, and as the process by which this state of affairs is created and maintained' (Mullender and Ward 1993: 148).

A number of black women writers, in highlighting their personal experiences, demonstrate the interacting effects of gender and race (hooks 1981, 1989; Lorde 1984; Jordan 1989). Their writings provide rich sources of information about the effects of multiple oppression. The oppression of the individual is grounded in the beliefs and practice of a sexist, homophobic, disabilist, ageist, racist and class ridden society. Emma Goldman succinctly shows how the personal experiences of oppression and the structures that determine and maintain that oppression are linked when she states: 'it is organized violence at the top that permits individual violence at the bottom' (Weick and Vandiver 1982: 9).

Our experiences of oppression will mean that we have internalized what it means to be different and will therefore use that knowledge when we relate to others. This point is picked up by Lorde (1984: 122) who, in sharing her experiences of oppression as a woman, said that 'as women, we must root out internalised patterns of oppression within ourselves if we are to move beyond the most superficial aspects of social change'. It is also necessary to examine where the power which produces and sustains specific forms of powerlessness is located. This can only be done, however, if we accept the interconnectedness as well as the specificity of each named oppression. It is only by addressing these points that it is possible to combat oppression effectively.

Interconnections

Often we label people and put them into boxes like good/bad, deserving/undeserving and so on. This focus on dichotomy leads to 'forced choices, to unnecessary competition, and to unequal relationships in which one half of the pair is viewed as inferior and the other as superior' (Kolb-Morris 1993: 101). However, it is important to view human life from a holistic perspective. Difference should be seen as a source of strength and power.

A black feminist perspective attempts to address this issue of difference. It argues that oppression should not be ranked, or compartmentalized, but that the interconnectedness of oppressions should be emphasized. It is only through the making of such links that a true understanding of how oppression structures an individual's life can be obtained. bell hooks makes this point clearly. In reflecting upon her experiences of, and involvement in, feminist struggle, she writes: 'at the moment of my birth, two factors determined my destiny, my having been born black and my having been born female' (hooks 1981: 12). Both black women and white women therefore need to take into account the following points if they are to engage effectively in the process of change:

- to end the oppression of black women, both sexism and racism have to be addressed;
- to separate racism and sexism is to deny a basic truth of black women's existence.

Oppression can be specific in that it is manifested in one form or another, such as racism, sexism, heterosexism, disabilism, adultism and so on. But these forms also interconnect. The important point is that one aspect of ourselves should not be used to define the whole of us, as this is 'destructive and fragmenting' (Lorde 1984: 120).

A framework for theory and practice

The dual perspective informs our thinking, our work, and relationships with other people. Together with an understanding of power and oppression it can provide us with a framework within which to operate based on:

- personal self-knowledge;
- knowledge and an understanding of the majority social systems;
- knowledge and understanding of different groups and cultures;
- knowledge of how to challenge and confront issues on a personal and structural level;
- awareness of the need to be 'research minded' (Everitt *et al.* 1992);
- commitment to action and change.

These six points, together with an understanding of power and oppression, contribute to the development of anti-oppressive practice. The framework enables links to be made between individual action and social structures. It informs practice by enabling the worker to evaluate differences that exist at an individual level and within society and how these impact on each other. It provides the means of making accurate assessments by taking account of the inequalities that texture the lives of those denied access to society's resources because of their defined social status and the exclusionary practices of the dominant system. It demands that we constantly engage in the process of critical self-examination, which in turn enables us to engage in the process of change.

Change – which, we would argue, should be central to a practice that is anti-oppressive – is rooted in people's lived experiences. It is important that our work and interactions with others make a difference, not only to their lives but to our own. It is vital when working with people who are oppressed that change takes place. The task of anti-oppressive practice is to span the gulf that exists between what we feel and think and our ability to take control of our lives. Anti-oppressive practice makes clear the links that exist between our inner *subjective* world and the external world.

If we are to combat oppression we need first to *understand* the mechanisms that result in people being denied access to resources, and thus feeling powerless. Secondly, we must try to *provide the means* by which individuals can regain control of their lives. The law can be seen as a vehicle for change. As a source of power, it is a structure which can direct people's practice. But more importantly it is people's practice that can transform it into a radical tool. If we regard the law as a resource that has the potential to enhance our practice, then we hold the key to change. The law has to be seen as a *process*, not just a structure that has its own reality. But it is a process that we can engage in and use for the purpose of empowering others.

Linking theory and practice

For health and social care practitioners and carers it is important to understand the realities of the lives of those we work with and care for. An understanding of how oppressed groups can harness the power of their experiences to challenge the prevailing social relations enables us as practitioners and carers to develop a positive practice. It is not easy to take action against the structures of oppression – it involves 'hard intellectual and emotional work' (Watt and Cook 1993: 133), a challenge that has to be taken up.

In order to illustrate how the challenge can be taken up, we will consider a study which looked at the experiences of black women social workers (Burke 1990). Through their experiences the study sought to discover what strategies black women social workers were able to develop in order to promote anti-racist and anti-sexist practice. The data collected provided evidence of the strengths of those who are engaged in the struggle against racism and sexism. As we consider the research study in more detail, reflect upon these points and consider how research minded practitioners can engage in the task of critically analysing their own positions.

Everitt and her co-writers (1992: 134) discuss the importance of using research methodologies in order to 'develop new kinds of critical reflective practice'. The need for 'research mindedness' is reflected in our framework for theory and practice, as is the importance of critical analysis. Everitt *et al.* (1992: 134) suggest a number of particular ways of thinking about theory and practice, including:

- questioning taken-for-granted assumptions about the definition of problems and categorization of need;
- recognizing the ways in which ideas, thoughts, understandings and opinions are shaped historically, economically, politically and socially through social structures and processes;
- making the implicit explicit;
- raising the profile of value positions and working with the problematics they generate;
- locating practice in its agency contexts so that service delivery issues are not addressed as routine constraints;
- building reflection, involvement and evaluation into every stage of the practice process.

We began this chapter with a consideration of the personal reality of people's lives and the structural context of those lives. This study took as its starting point the reality of black women's lives within a social services department. The research was undertaken by a black woman using participatory and feminist research techniques. The researcher was concerned not to neglect or objectify the women in the research process. The researcher therefore shared and explored with the women involved their experiences of oppression in a social services department. From that informed dialogue the researcher was able to identify strategies that the women had developed and were using to promote change. The study provided evidence of how sexism and racism determined the working lives of black professional women. It also demonstrated how these professional workers overcame the resistance of the social service structures and actively engaged in anti-oppressive practice.

The information obtained from interviewing 24 women social care practitioners indicated that the black women on a personal level were utilizing their experience of struggle to inform their practice. They managed, in an environment that did not promote race and sex equality, to develop and engage in anti-oppressive practice. The nurturing and support received from friends, family and communities enabled the women to counteract their experiences of not feeling valued and being disempowered. This positive experience informed their own practice, a practice which was in opposition to accepted practices and was empowering to service users.

The women in the study developed a number of strategies which enabled them to continue to work from an anti-oppressive perspective in the face of personal and structural challenges. We view these strategies as *nurturing*, for they sustain the individual and counteract the negative effects of racial and sexual oppression. Operating from a dual perspective the women did not locate the sources of dysfunction within themselves. They looked for the existence of structural barriers that the dominant system had erected against them. The women were armed with the knowledge, values and aspirations gained from the smaller system (i.e. friends, families, communities), and an understanding of the socio-economic and political barriers erected by the larger dominant system (of which the social services department is a microcosm). This enabled them to challenge and confront issues and develop strategies aimed at removing those barriers and promoting anti-oppressive practice. The strategies are as follows:

1 *Working collectively with other black colleagues* and those committed to working from an anti-racist, anti-sexist perspective. By working collectively the individual experiences of oppression and ways of combating oppression could be pooled together. Collective working also provided the opportunity for supportive networks to be developed.
2 *The setting of achievable tasks* enabled the black women to address effectively the issues of oppression. They were able to focus and channel their energies. They had to set realistic goals if they were to bring about change. The setting of realistic goals meant that the women were able to focus and channel their energies and so effectively bring about change.
3 *Utilizing existing policies and legislation* as tools to combat oppression.
4 *Being informed.* It is essential that workers consolidate their personal experiences of oppression within a wider theoretical and political framework. It is also important that workers have knowledge and understanding of issues that have direct or indirect implications for themselves as practitioners and for service users.
5 *Strategic positioning* in order to influence change and become part of the change process. It is important for practitioners to achieve power not just at the grass roots level but at the various levels of the hierarchy.
6 *Being strong and positive in the face of adversity.* The adoption of this philosophy provided the impetus for the black women to continue in their struggles in spite of personal experiences of oppression.

This research contributes to the development of anti-oppressive theory. It demonstrates how, out of the experiences of oppression and powerlessness, strategies for change can be developed. The research thus provides us with evidence of how change can and does occur and how people have used their experiences to change and inform policy and practice.

Final thoughts

The use of the dual perspective enables us to locate an individual's personal experiences of oppression within the context of her or his social environment. It enables us to evaluate our own value position in relation to others and thus to take account of differences and similarities. It helps us to understand powerlessness and through this the nature of power within society. We end this chapter with the following personal account, which portrays the ideas, thoughts and feelings contained in the chapter.

> In my interactions with other people, which can be in formal and informal settings – the workplace, at home, attending a conference, eating out at a restaurant, through discussion or heated argument, in the role of helper or being helped – I am guided, like us all, by the ideas that I have about the total system in which we all live. These ideas and thoughts may not always be systematic, orthodox or stand up to empirical testing. But they are informed by my lived experience. They allow me a window from which I can view and understand my relationship with the world I live in. As a black woman I recognize that black and white women have different histories and that the power relations that exist between them are complex and real. The impact and consequence of oppression, which is manifested in a number of ways, deconstructs the idea that we all share a common experience. Oppression makes our lives distinctive and separate, but it also enables us to understand what we have in common. My experience as a black woman working within white organizations not only provides me with a continual and rich source of information which enables me to develop an understanding of how social relations between people (be they black or white, male or female etc.) are played out. But also demonstrates how those subject to the forces of oppression positively and actively combat them.

We began with a personal account of Chrissie's experiences as a young person in residential care; we finished with a personal account of the experiences of a black woman. We drew a distinction in the introduction between anti-oppressive and anti-discriminatory practice. Before moving on, perhaps you would now like to reflect on this chapter and think about the differences and what they mean to you. You may also wish to document your own experiences of power, powerlessness and oppression to assist you in this process.

2 USING LEGISLATION –

A LIBERAL OR RADICAL

APPROACH?

> The crisis in the law concerns an institution which is incapable or unwilling to adapt to a different order: a system unable to recognise its own failings. I hope I have demonstrated that while the law is in a lamentable state it can be changed; it can be challenged and is being reformed to some degree.
>
> (Helena Kennedy 1993: 264)

Every day, practitioners are engaged in the practice of listening to individuals, communicating with someone, ensuring that service users can access welfare services. We are all involved in the human activity of living. In Chapter 1 we explored how living can be understood in terms of interconnections. This living is informed by contractual obligations, duties and responsibilities. Working within the welfare state we, as members of the caring professions or as carers, are bound by the legislative framework. We are not experts in law, but we have to have a working knowledge of the legislation if we are to utilize it effectively. Knowledge is not just about what the law states, it is about being able to understand the problems and dilemmas that we come across in our day-to-day work and it is about being able to think through these difficulties and find solutions to them.

This chapter looks at why we have chosen to use the vehicle of the law to promote anti-oppressive practice. We will consider the contradictions and dilemmas that are present in the law, which mean that it can be seen as constraining and oppressive or can be used as a radical tool.

The law is not usually the first resort in our interactions with others, but it is available to us – like an artist's palette, visible to the eye, potentially to be used. Application of the law demands from us a number of skills. For it to be available we have to know what it states and be able to apply it to the different situations that we encounter.

Some commentators have argued that the law is not an instrument that can be used to promote anti-oppressive practice. 'The legal powers and remedies available . . . do not always empower them to protect vulnerable people' (Braye and Preston-Shoot 1992a: 3). It is seen as a 'blunt instrument' (Brayne and Martin 1990: 287) designed not to enhance people's positions but to maintain them. To take the law on is often seen as an arduous, thankless task (Braye and Preston-Shoot 1992a: 3; Vernon 1993: 2). We would agree. Yet the law can be harnessed, it can be changed and it can be used to benefit and empower. However, it has to be used with this point of view in mind.

The debate

Andy and Charlie are two practitioners who have views concerning their use of the legal authority invested in them. Charlie is trying to convince her colleague that the law can be used positively to promote change. The debate reflects their principles, their knowledge and their application of the law in relation to health and social care practice.

Andy: How can you possibly write about anti-oppressive practice and the law when everyone knows that the law is based on maintaining things as they are?

Charlie: I can understand what you're saying but the law doesn't have to be about state control – I see it as something that can be used to promote change and used as a positive resource to promote good practice.

Andy: I find that difficult to believe. Look at the Race Relations Act: the first person to be prosecuted was a black man. You're telling me that that's good practice?

Charlie: Of course not. But what I am thinking about is a wider debate than just looking at anti-discriminatory legislation. It is about looking at how legal intervention can be used to promote good practice. After all, there is no getting away from the fact that we have to work within a legal framework.

Andy: Yes, but we've got no control over that.

Charlie: But we do have control over how we use legislation in promoting the rights of people we work with and care for.

Andy: I just don't see how you and I can use the law as a means of promoting change. It's difficult enough for some of the campaigning groups like Family Rights Group, MIND or the disability forums to do it.

Charlie: Yes, but you are saying that the law is very powerful. Surely you can see that we can harness that power to make it work for us?

Andy: As far as I'm concerned as a practitioner I'll do everything I can to avoid using the law. I hate going to court – if I can possibly get out of it I will. All I can see it doing in my work is monitoring parents, in fact monitoring mothers: discriminating against them and labelling them as 'inadequate'. It's just oppressive and controlling.

Charlie: Yes, the law is complex and can be contradictory. And I don't like going to court either, but I blame our training for that: we talked about theory and we learned about what legislation we might need to use but we were never really taught how to use the law in practice. But as practitioners we have to question the moral dilemmas that face us and understand how the law can help us get through them and not see the law as an obstruction. Surely if we know the law and understand it then we can get it to work for us rather than against us?

Andy: Well *you* might think you can get it to work for you but I don't see how *I* can.

Charlie: OK. Take the case of Danny – he used to have meals on wheels at home but then got himself a part-time job. So he asked for the meals to be delivered to his workplace. They wouldn't do that because they couldn't afford to re-route to take in the workplace. The home care organizer became involved and it was agreed that two frozen meals for the days that Danny was at work would be delivered at the beginning of the week.

Andy: Well, his situation must have got better if he had a job – only people who are housebound should get meals on wheels anyway.

Charlie: Not at all. The need was still the same because the assessment was based on the fact that cooking was dangerous and difficult for him because of his disability, which left his arms weak. The issue here is that the assessment and service offered was focused on keeping him in a position of dependency instead of enabling him to maintain his independence within the community. Under the 1986 Disabled Persons Act a comprehensive assessment of Danny's needs was made. A change in circumstances didn't change his needs. Social services have a duty to meet any assessed need for services which fall under Section 2 of the 1970 Chronically Sick and Disabled Persons Act. Financial constraints do not affect the statutory obligation to meet these needs. The home care organizer, having made the initial assessment, recognized the importance for Danny of maintaining his independence and also that they had a duty to provide him with a service. She therefore used the law creatively despite resource constraints, to ensure that Danny had a meal and kept his dignity and independence. It was actually better than delivering it to the workplace, but when Danny first made the request that seemed the logical solution. The home care organizer not only worked in partnership with him but was not going to be defeated at the first hurdle. She was very much in tune with a needs-led approach which ultimately means independence.

Andy: Right, I am beginning to understand your point of view. I obviously need to think a bit more about anti-oppressive practice.

The above dialogue demonstrates the contradictions, dilemmas and tensions that characterize the uneasy relationship which appears to exist between practitioners, users and the legislative framework. Andy's perspective is typical of that of many workers, whose view of the law is one of ambivalence or hostility. He sees the law as unclear, unhelpful, punitive in its impact and constraining – in short a 'necessary evil'. He feels powerless as a worker against the weight of the legislative process, which he does not understand. He feels its purposes are often contradictory and this contributes to his own role ambiguity (Braye and Preston-Shoot 1992a). Charlie recognizes the complex relationship that exists between the legal framework and the objectives of social work intervention. Her competence is demonstrated by her ability to integrate relevant legislation, policy and procedures into her practice, and she has been able to evaluate these critically in relation to the anti-oppressive values she holds. She has used the law creatively to challenge oppression and powerlessness (Lee 1991). Such discussions will continue, however, as Morris and Nott (1991: 193) point out:

> There will always be debate between those who are sceptical about the power of the law to change society and those whose legal training makes them reluctant to acknowledge the law's limitations or to dismiss the law entirely.

Value perspectives and the law

Legislation is the primary political instrument for bringing about social and economic change. The law is also a central element of social care practice. However, it can be argued that legislation is oppressive and disempowering to service users. If anti-oppressive practice is fundamentally about change, then it could be argued that the law is limiting in the way in which it can bring about real change in society. As April Carter (1988: 140) points out,

> ingrained attitudes based on historical social practices do change only slowly, and therefore laws may promote lip service to the principle of equal treatment and token gestures towards implementing it, without resulting in any fundamental alterations in the economic and social structures of society.

At one level campaigns for legislation have been the central focus for various pressure groups representing marginalized groups in society (children, women, gays and lesbians, single parents, etc.) who have fought hard for statutes to improve their position. At another level such groups have often been disappointed by the results of legislation and this has led to a cynical questioning of the effectiveness of the law in promoting anti-oppressive practice. For example, the Sex Discrimination Act 1975 has been criticized as being only of value as a declaration of intent rather than making a significant difference to the lives of women by being a radical measure to change individuals' behaviour (a similar criticism is made about other anti-discrimination legislation).

The power of the law, however, must not be underestimated. In discussing the use of legislation to improve the position of women in society, Morris and Nott (1991: 11) argue against those who repudiate the law as a means of promoting change and suggest that 'if the law is so powerful, it should be possible to harness that power to the cause of women and thus use the law as a positive force'. They go on to state that although this may not be easy to achieve, understanding the law is the first process towards using it. All too often health and social care practitioners, and carers, find the law difficult, confusing and an 'obstacle to practice' (Braye and Preston-Shoot 1992a: 3) and choose to consider that it is not necessary either to understand the law or to use it appropriately. They point to the fact that the institutional systems within which the law operates are, of themselves, oppressive and function to maintain the power structures within society. There is of course some truth in this and it is therefore necessary to understand some analysis of the purpose of legislation.

Given that we have to work within the framework of the law, we also have to appreciate the fact that it is not value free, but is shaped by social, political, historical and economic factors. Suzy Braye and Michael Preston-Shoot (1992a: 15) reiterate this point when they state that in practice, the law 'is far from being a value free activity and cannot be negotiated by reference merely to technical knowledge'. It has been said that there is a contradiction between the law in books and the law in action (McBarnet 1981). Various writers have demonstrated that there are a number of myths surrounding the institutions which purport to do justice; that is, the institutions of the judiciary, the magistrates and the courts. Gifford (1986) discusses the myth that we have the 'finest legal system in the world', based on the impartiality of the judiciary. Griffiths (1977: 219) talks about the myth of neutrality, suggesting that neither impartiality nor independence involve neutrality. Griffiths also suggests that 'one of the greatest political myths' is that the courts are for the individual and against the power of the state.

We have then, as McBarnet (1981) demonstrates, a gap between the law and the rhetoric of justice which exists because it functions within an authoritarian state. The significance of law is that not only does it consist of rules for criminal justice, it is also the means by which the state rules. Governments make these rules and without them they would be unable to function. Governments also represent stability and have an interest in preserving that stability and maintaining authoritarian structures in public institutions – thus while governments might be controlled by the courts, the judiciary is essentially a part of the governing group and thus will operate to maintain the system rather than have regard for the individual. As Braye and Preston-Shoot (1993: 16) point out,

> The law preserves the status quo within the power structures of society. Whilst predicated upon the rhetoric of freedom, justice and equality, the law colludes with inequalities between women and men, black people and white people, people with disabilities and able-bodied people, young and old.

Using the law to promote good practice

The functions of the law can be seen to have contradictory elements, but we would argue that the law can offer the opportunity to promote good practice. Moreover, bearing in mind that we have to work within a statutory framework, it is important to manage this from an anti-oppressive perspective. In discussing the reasons for passing laws to forbid discrimination, Carter (1988) argues that the purpose of legislation is to change attitudes, influence behaviour, give moral backing to those who wish to practise equal treatment and provide the means of enforcing a change in social and economic practices.

If we now take this point and relate it to the Children Act 1989 we can see that the Act has already changed attitudes and practice in a number of areas.

Children's and young people's rights

People are becoming aware of the need to respect and value the views of young people and to involve them in the decision making processes concerning their lives. Health and social care practitioners who are concerned to promote the rights of children and young people are now able to refer to substantive law to support their practice. Indeed, many local authorities are recognizing the need to ensure that the rights of young people are not denied or violated, by appointing children's rights officers.

Listening to the views of young people

Another area where practice is improving is in the taking of instructions from children and young people by solicitors. King and Young (1993) have discussed some of the practice issues in relation to ensuring that the views of young people are respected. They point out that the case of a child or young person is rarely clear cut and young people may face dilemmas when giving instructions. They therefore advise that it is helpful to consider the least damaging option and that the flexibility of the Children Act 1989 means there are various orders to which conditions can be attached, which may have different effects. Thus they suggest that if a guardian *ad litem* wishes to recommend an order of a certain kind but the young person does not agree, an imaginative solicitor could produce a menu of orders which both parties could accept.

While social workers may need to know the law as well as lawyers, they can also work together with lawyers to ensure that the law is used imaginatively and effectively so that the rights of the young person are respected. Practice therefore may not be perfect in relation to young people, but it is certainly improving as a consequence of the legislation.

Secure accommodation

At the other end of the spectrum the law is identified by practitioners as something which has to be 'embraced uncritically, as it offers certainty and direction in an uncertain and confusing world' (Braye and Preston-Shoot 1992a: 3). Consider the law regarding secure accommodation for young people, which has been described as 'chameleon-like provision' (Harris and Timms 1993b: 24). As well as being used for Section 53 orders or to ensure young people's own protection, it can also be used strategically to keep them out of the criminal justice system. The use of secure accommodation reflects the tensions between the principles of protecting children, protecting the community and protecting ourselves as workers. These tensions are reflected in the conflicting philosophies underpinning the Children Act 1989 and the Criminal Justice Act 1991.

In order to reduce inappropriate use of secure accommodation, Harris and Timms (1993a) focus on the practice of social workers rather than on any technical change in legislation or the expectation that the courts will make the appropriate decision. They suggest a number of ways in which social workers can effectively use the current legislation to ensure that orders are made which are appropriate to the needs of the child or young person. These include:

- examination of the agency's gatekeeping policies;
- consideration of the length of time that an order is needed (i.e. orders do not have to be for the maximum duration);
- ensuring that the order is made within the framework of a clear plan for the child;
- rigorous departmental scrutiny preceding renewal applications, so that the court does not just rubber stamp them and so endorse unplanned practice.

One of their research findings indicated that most courts were unwilling to turn down applications from expert professionals. Therefore it is not enough for social workers to rely on the legislation or the courts to solve the problems presented by the differing uses of secure accommodation orders. Nor should they assume that court hearings remove the responsibility for decision making from them in difficult child care cases. In the 'uncertain and confusing' world of juvenile justice legislation social workers should not 'embrace uncritically' the decisions made by the courts. As Harris and Timms (1993a) point out, the role of the social worker is crucial in determining the outcome of court decisions.

Race and culture issues

In dealing with young people from a variety of cultural and ethnic backgrounds it is important that health and social care practitioners have a good understanding of the Children Act 1989 and are familiar with the provisions of the Race Relations Act 1976. Staff should also be aware of and sensitive to the background of the young people. They should be able to communicate their understanding effectively and provide a service that is anti-racist and anti-oppressive in its impact.

It is often a difficult task for health and social care practitioners to assess exactly what the *wishes and feelings* of a young person might be, but it is an essential requirement of the Act. Historically, the feelings and needs of black young people have not been adequately assessed and may even be disregarded. Failure to address their wishes and feelings (and thus their needs) has had a punitive effect on black children (Barn 1983; Ahmed *et al.* 1986).

The primary aim of the Act is that 'the child's welfare shall be the court's paramount consideration' (Section 1(1)). While 'welfare' is not defined, this must include considering the race, religion, culture and language of the child. The welfare checklist (Section 1(3)) which a court shall have regard to does assist, however, and this is headed by the requirement that 'the ascertainable wishes and feelings of the child concerned' (Section 1(3)(a)) must be considered. Often young people are struggling to find their identity within their own changing cultures in this country. It is therefore essential for health and social care practitioners to be able to understand the complexities of various cultures, which all have their own internal dynamics. In discussing the Children Act 1989 we have noted that its potential will only be realized if it is imaginatively used by committed anti-racist workers. Real change with regard to the needs of black children will need to be monitored, but it is only when opportunities that the Act presents are implemented that the situation for black children will change (Burke and Dalrymple 1991).

Let us take the example of black care leavers to illustrate this. Research by CHAR (McCluskey 1993) has identified that black care leavers are a high risk group, and vulnerable to homelessness, despite the well documented duties of social services departments under the Children Act 1989. But the Act does provide opportunities to improve the situation for black care leavers by the principles of interagency collaboration (Sections 27, 28, 30 on housing and social services) and the need for specific care plans, which should not only incorporate support for care leavers but also consider the race, religion, culture and language of the young person.

Rights – whose rights are they?

Whoever we are we have rights. There are those of us who may feel that our rights are denied – perhaps some more than others. Rights have been described as 'valuable commodities' (Wasserstrom 1964: 628; quoted in Freeman 1983: 33), 'important moral coinage' (Freeman 1983: 33) or, concerning legal rights 'indispensably valuable possessions' (Feinberg 1966: 1; quoted in Freeman 1983: 33). There are, however, a number of distinctions which it will be useful to explore briefly.

First, it is important to recognize that there are basic universal rights, like those enshrined in documents such as the Universal Declaration of Human Rights. But one can also identify different kinds of rights, i.e. legal, social and civil rights. The concept of legal rights themselves can be considered in two ways: substantive and procedural rights. Basically, substantive rights can be understood as rights which give individuals power, enforceable by law, to take action to protect their own interests. Procedural rights ensure fairness in the decision making process.

King and Trowell (1992) suggest that the promotion of children's rights through use of the law or legal intervention is not as straightforward as it might seem. In child abuse cases parents may be prosecuted or imprisoned without consideration of the children involved, or the children may be removed from home, again without regard to their wishes and feelings. In their critique, they suggest that when these matters are discussed with children, it is not always easy to know *how much* they should be involved. In this way workers fail to appreciate that working from an anti-oppressive perspective requires one to consider the rights of children, which are backed up by the legislation in the Children Act 1989. The issue for us is not how *much* children should be involved but *how*.

While the term 'rights' is not itself included in the Act, it does 'represent significant advances for the capacity of children to contribute to . . . decisions affecting their future' (Frost 1992: 9) and it is informed by a rights based ideology. One of the value positions informing the Act is that of children's rights and child liberation (Fox-Harding 1991) and there are a number of duties which clearly indicate that those involved in working with children must ensure their maximum involvement in the decision making (e.g. Sections 1, 22, 26). Within the development of social care practice, relationships within families which are considered to be in the private domain become public concerns. For instance, informal care of vulnerable people that springs 'from personal ties of kinship, friendship and neighbourhood' (DHSS 1981) has been formalized by the Community Care legislation. However, consideration of issues of rights within the private domain can be problematic (Ungerson 1993). One of the arguments that Ungerson puts forward is that within the family unequal power relationships exist. Therefore a number of difficulties exist around the area of caring:

> do children have a right to their parents', or more particularly, their mothers' continual attention? Do parents, once they have grown frail and elderly, have a right to be cared for by their children and the right to be financially maintained by their better-off kin? Do people deemed to be schizophrenic have a right to be looked after by their parents, or, conversely, a right not to be looked after by their parents?
>
> (Ungerson 1993: 144)

One element of anti-oppressive practice is to ensure that people's rights are not violated. In terms of anti-oppressive practice and the law it is important to understand how rights are enshrined within the legislation as well as to recognize how it can be said to deny people their rights. We need to be aware of our role in ensuring that minimizing the oppressive aspects of such legislation serves to maximize the rights to which they are entitled.

How do we do this? It is not always easy. Should a woman with diabetes, prone to regular comas, be allowed to live alone with her baby? Should an 80-year-old woman who has refused a home care assessment, following admission to hospital after being severely bruised at the hands of her husband, be allowed home? You are aware that she has suffered a lifetime of abuse but now she is too frail to cope.

These both pose moral and ethical practice dilemmas in which a worker or carer could choose to use the law to deny the right to be a parent, or to deny the right to refuse a service. Alternatively we could use the legislation to protect and balance the rights of all those involved. In the case of the diabetic mother, the philosophy of the Children Act 1989 is that the child should be brought up in her or his own family and that the local authority should work in partnership with the parent(s) to provide a range of services appropriate to that child's needs (Volume 2 Guidance and Regulations on the 1989 Children Act). The child has a right to family life and a right to protection (Braye and Preston-Shoot 1993). The mother has a right to parental autonomy but not the right to endanger the life of her child should she go into a coma and thus leave the child without adequate care.

In the case of the older woman the decision to use compulsory powers to protect her from further abuse could be made under the general powers of the Mental Health Act 1983 or Section 47 of the National Assistance Act 1948. However, this demonstrates the 'messiness' of ethical problems concerning older people (Stevenson 1989) and judgements about degree of risk to the person concerned. Arguments about the duty to care versus minimal intervention are not easy to address. However, the assessment should be undertaken in conjunction with the service user. What has happened is that the home care facility has been used as a way of 'monitoring' the situation without consultation with the person concerned. Thus it is a response to the needs of the professionals to protect her rather than to her needs for a service. In this way the use of legislation could be said to be oppressive. An assessment completed in partnership with the person concerned could be used as a system of 'social support' which offers choices to the user, rather than of 'social control' which merely offers solutions (DoH Care Management and Assessment: Practitioners Guide).

Obligations

Fifteen-year-old Veronica is pregnant to John, who is known to be involved in a male prostitution ring. They share a house together and the relationship is important to her. Although she is aware of his sexual activities, she believes that within the relationship her needs are being met. Her social worker is concerned that the relationship is abusive and that she is being exploited. She feels that she has a legal obligation to protect Veronica and is considering using the child care legislation to deny her continuing in this relationship. This course of action causes a number of dilemmas for the social worker.

The social worker is aware of how much the relationship with John means to Veronica. Veronica is pregnant, needs a lot of support and considers that John meets her emotional needs. Veronica can be considered to be 'Gillick competent', and is therefore able to make her own choices and has a right to do so. The worker has a good relationship with Veronica and has tried to give her as much information as possible about her concerns should Veronica remain in the house. After some discussion about the options available to Veronica the social worker decided that recourse to the law was the only alternative left if Veronica's identified needs were to be met. Veronica was eventually moved to foster carers where she subsequently was able to reflect on the situation. She eventually ceased further contact with John of her own volition.

An obligation can be understood as a morally binding relationship between individuals based on reciprocal biographies. We all feel obligations at various times to various people. At times such obligations can be competing and we have to make choices (Finch and Mason 1990; Jordan 1990). What choices did Veronica have? She had a relationship with John which she felt was satisfactory. But through her social worker she had access to information which made her question that relationship. The social worker through her work with Veronica had access to information about John. She also had an understanding of the risks that Veronica and the unborn child faced. In giving her information the social worker tried to assist Veronica to make choices. The social worker had a legal obligation to ensure that Veronica's wishes and feelings were taken into account, to consider her physical and emotional needs and any harm she was likely to suffer.

The social worker faced dilemmas in terms of anti-oppressive practice. Was it best to intervene now, or to intervene in a more oppressive manner at a later stage? She felt immediate intervention was best. It was preferable to leaving Veronica in her current situation, where she would be further exploited and abused. This would only result in more oppressive action being taken as further evidence of potential dangers emerged. The worker therefore felt that she had a moral obligation to protect Veronica and the baby and used the law to facilitate this, having also fulfilled her obligations to involve Veronica completely in the decision making process and keep her informed throughout that process.

Duties

A duty, imposed by statute, has to be carried out. There is no choice in this and however difficult it might be to do there is no acceptable reason for not doing so. Sometimes people confuse duties and powers. A power is something which statute gives to individuals or bodies but they can choose whether or not to exercise that power – there is no obligation to do so. It is the imposition of duties which people in social care practice may feel contributes to the oppressive elements of legislation. However, a duty can also be a powerful force in promoting rights and ensuring adequate provision of services – lack of money is not a good enough reason for not carrying out a duty, for instance. So if a service is not provided because a local authority states that there is not enough money in the budget then it is acting illegally.

The law and anti-oppressive practice

The mother of 11-year-old Zenab suffers from a psychotic illness. Zenab was placed in a foster home after her mother experienced a psychotic episode and was then unable to seek medical treatment for Zenab. The foster carer, from talking to her and from her play and drawings, became aware that while Zenab said that she wanted to go home she also indicated that she felt unsure about this. Zenab clearly had a good relationship with her mother but at times, when her mother was ill, she became unhappy and this made her anxious about a possible return home. The social worker also recognized the confusion felt by Zenab. In the foster home her physical health and school performance improved considerably. The mother continued to suffer from psychotic episodes and required regular hospital admissions.

Andy and Charlie continue their debate by discussing Zenab's situation:

Andy: I thought anti-oppressive practice was about listening to the child. If you'd listened to Zenab you'd have let her go home to her Mum and that would probably have meant that she'd finish up suffering and damaged for ever.

Charlie: Yes, anti-oppressive practice is about listening to the child, but it is also about knowing your own value base which informs how you work with people. I am committed to an anti-oppressive practice perspective and empowering people with whom I work. So that means taking account of the context, listening and respecting Zenab's confusion and working to help her through that. It's about making a full assessment without making assumptions – for instance, just because she's doing well with the foster carers doesn't mean she wants to stay there for life. It just means that they have the resources that her mother doesn't currently have to look after Zenab. We have to take account of the mother's resources in view of her mental health.

Andy: Well, as far as I'm concerned my primary consideration would be Zenab and her welfare would be paramount. So if she's doing well with the carers, my assessment would be to leave her there and find her a permanent substitute family. Too many foster carers do a good job and all their good work is undone because some social worker comes along and decides the child should go home.

Charlie: That's typical of someone who wants a rehabilitation plan to fail. People like you should be taken to court for not doing your job properly! My assessment would be that if Zenab is confused it could well be that it is because she does really want to live with her Mum but that she wants it to be OK. Also, it's important to take account of issues about 'race' – is this an appropriate long-term placement? And equally important is the welfare of the mother and her wishes and feelings.

Andy: Well, she's psychotic isn't she? She's in and out of hospital like a yo-yo: what views could she possibly have that are going to be worthwhile? I don't mean to be difficult but let's be realistic.

Charlie: Look, she's looked after Zenab for a long time. They have a good relationship. We need to consider the times when she's well and look at supporting her – which you could do under Part III of the Children Act 1989. She has parental responsibility and has a right to be involved in any decisions about Zenab's life. It is up to us to work with her.

Andy: So you're telling me that you have an obligation to ascertain the wishes of the mother as well as Zenab? What about your professional assessment?

Charlie: Just because I'm a professional doesn't mean my views should override everyone else's. I have to take responsibility for the views I express and the judgements that I make, and I'd rather do this in partnership with everyone involved – the foster carer, the Mum and Zenab.

Andy: Well, maybe the carer thinks that Zenab shouldn't go home.

Charlie: If that's the case then her views also have to be listened to – it's about making a decision which takes everyone's views into account and it may be that my view is not the accepted view. What is important is that everyone has been involved in that process and a plan is made which everyone understands is the right way forward. I agree with you that we need to develop a solution which isn't oppressive to the Mum, but the solution also needs to protect Zenab's welfare. We have at least three lots of legislation to which we can refer to try and do that – there's the Children Act 1989, the NHS and Community Care Act 1990 and the Mental Health Act 1983.

Final thoughts

Andy doesn't see the law in an enlightened way. He chooses to use it as a means to an end which could be oppressive to both Zenab and her mother. He may genuinely believe that he is working in the best interests of the child, i.e. from a liberal traditional perspective. Charlie, on the other hand, is incorporating the best interests of Zenab in her practice but is aware of the rights of all the individuals involved and so from her perspective uses the law to enable a more radical approach to her practice.

Michael Freeman (1992: 4) has reminded us that 'legislation is a political act with political consequences, using political language and political symbols'. Our knowledge, values, theories and skills provide the framework which informs our practice. To use it in a radical way we have to acknowledge its weaknesses and harness its strengths.

Part II A MODEL OF

ANTI-OPPRESSIVE PRACTICE:

PRINCIPLES FOR ACTION

3   VALUES

Conservative

Conservative,
What does it mean?
Is it a swear word, or is it obscene?
I asked my mum,
But she wouldn't tell,
And then my dad and he said,
'Well . . .',
'A conservative man is a man with money,
He's top class and never funny,
He's like Robin Hood in reverse,
Taking money from the housewives' purse.'

The very next day,
As I passed by the shops,
Where I saw Mum paying Mr. Potts,
I ran in and shouted,
'You conservative man . . .
And Mum don't you ever pay that man!'
                    (Christopher Richard Kwaku Kyem 1994)

The way in which we consider legislation and whether we feel that it can be used as a liberal or radical tool is informed by our personal value base. It is important to have an understanding that legislation is value-laden and to know what our own value base is. We also need to be aware that our personal biographies will affect that value base and will continue to affect it as we are exposed to different influences. In this chapter we will explore how it is possible to use legislation effectively in a way which promotes anti-oppressive practice. We will begin this process with a consideration of where the value base of the law is located – bearing in mind that it is a 'political act', as we were reminded at the end of Chapter 2. We will then go on to consider how we locate ourselves and how we can work within the legislative framework to tip the balance from oppressive to anti-oppressive practice.

Value base of the law: where is it coming from?

When we first set out on this venture many of our friends and colleagues challenged our assumption that it was possible to use the law to promote anti-oppressive practice. The following statements encapsulate some of the points of view presented by others concerning the value base of the law:

> The law is inflexible and insensitive. It over-simplifies the difficult moral issues we have to try and deal with.
>
> The law merely adds to the dilemmas we face – it doesn't help us at all.
>
> How can the law support anti-oppressive practice when some areas of discrimination are still lawful?
>
> In total about 20 different points of law either explicitly or by omission discriminate against the lesbian and gay community. The end result is that homosexuals are officially relegated to a second class citizenship: denied equality in law and subject to institutional discrimination in virtually every aspect of our lives.
>
> (Tatchell 1992: 237)

The law is a set of legal rules. We discussed in the previous chapter the fact that it is governments who make these rules and that without them they would be unable to function. Governments also represent stability and maintenance of authoritarian structures in public institutions. Furthermore, the judiciary is essentially a part of the governing group and thus will operate to maintain the system. Therefore, it can be argued that the law functions: to preserve power structures (e.g. racist systems of social control as evidenced by the increased use of compulsory powers in admissions of young Afro-Caribbean men to psychiatric hospital); to act as an agent of social control (e.g. Section 28 of the Local Government Act 1988, which attempts to control homosexuality); to provide 'solutions' to social problems ('the Mental Health Act 1983 enables madness to be contained behind locked doors'); to further political ideology (e.g. the National Health Service and Community Care Act 1990 is underpinned by the ideology of market values and the mixed economy of care) (Braye and Preston-Shoot 1992a).

Let us just think about the value base of the law in more detail. A significant element in the philosophy of the Children Act 1989 is 'the belief that children are best looked after within the family with both parents playing a full part and without resort to legal proceedings' (HMSO 1993). While 'family' is rarely clearly defined in legislation there is the assumption – as indicated in the government publications concerning the Act – that it is a particular one: two married people, male and female, living together with two children of the marriage; the father as *breadwinner*, the mother as *carer*. The parents are expected to be responsible for the upbringing of the children to the degree that the children arguably might be considered to be the *property* of their parents.

Now we need to consider how such values might affect legislation.

Marriage

Although two people may live together and share the parenting of a child for a considerable number of years a cohabitee 'by no stretch of the imagination could . . . be described as a parent' (Children Act Advisory Committee 1992/3: 14). This was the conclusion in *Re J (a Minor: Property Transfer)* (1992) *The Times* 12 November, FD, where the question was whether the cohabitee of ten years' standing could properly be described as the parent of the child. While the word 'parent' can be used for a stepfather who has treated a child as the child of the family, a cohabitee who has never married the child's mother cannot be considered as a parent.

Within a relationship the couple must also be heterosexual. Thus although residence nearly always decides in favour of the mother, a mother who goes against this norm, i.e. a lesbian mother, is more likely to lose custody of her children. This is because 'A very material factor in considering where a child's welfare lies is which of two competing parents can offer the nearest approach to that norm' (in *Re C (a Minor)* reported in *The Guardian*, 17 October 1990).

Children as property

The Children Act has been hailed as a Children's Charter. While it does challenge the notion of children as the property of their parents, other legislation, such as the Education Act 1985, very much assumes that children are the property of their parents. Therefore all decisions concerning their education are made with parents (e.g. non school attendance, school exclusions). The Criminal Justice Act 1991 also introduced measures designed to increase levels of parental responsibility for their 'property'.

Parental responsibility

The term 'parental responsibility' is now on the statute books. Both the Children Act 1989 and the Child Support Act 1991 emphasize this concept and the government has stated that the two Acts should be seen as complementary pieces of legislation. However, commentators have noted that although the two may at first sight seem similar, under the Children Act the exercise of parental responsibility is comprehensive, while under the Child Support Act it is based purely in terms of finance. In effect the Child Support Act does not view working in partnership with parents as a viable option and holds that parents, particularly poor parents, cannot be trusted (Leigh 1992: 178).

It can therefore be seen, merely by looking briefly at the concept of the family, that there may be competing ideologies about what a 'family' might be. These ideologies inform legislation, which is also influenced by other ideologies. Some pieces of legislation may therefore conflict – which then leads to a lack of coherence. It is important therefore to understand the value base of the law as you go on to explore your own value base.

Being explicit about your own value base

Before we can start to think about working anti-oppressively within the law we need to locate ourselves. We can do this by thinking about our life and work experiences. From this we can start to build up a picture of who we are, where we are and why we feel that it is possible to work from an anti-oppressive perspective.

Sam's story

I am 15 years old and have been caring for my Dad for the last three years since my Mum died. My Dad always used to enjoy a drink but once Mum died he just seemed to get worse and worse. He lost his job and that didn't help matters. I really love my Dad and he was always great with me when I was younger. He would take me out; he'd always be there to watch me in the local football team; he always made me do my homework before I went out to meet my mates – which used to annoy me then – but I always did well in class in those days.

It's a bit difficult getting my homework done now because there's so much to do in the house. When I get home I often have to sort my Dad out. Sometimes he's flat out on the floor and so I have to get him up and if he's been sick there's that to clear up. There is always washing to be done because Dad just doesn't bother and often wets himself or is sick everywhere. Then I have to get myself something to eat. Often, by the time I've done all my jobs, I'm too tired to be starting on any homework. I think it's important to do well at school and Mum and Dad always encouraged me to do well. Sometimes I think I'm letting them down these days as I don't seem to get good marks and I'm sure I won't pass my exams.

Charmaine's story

I always knew I wanted to go into nursing – ever since I was little. I don't know why really, maybe it's because Auntie Edna was a nurse and I always got on well with her. My Mum always said that she didn't mind what I did when I left school as long as I got a good job. In nursing you meet a variety of people and even though they are sick you get to know them and it's good to be involved in caring for them. I get upset when someone on the ward dies – but you get over it soon enough because the bed is never empty for that long, and there is always someone else to care for. There have been quite a few changes over the years – there doesn't seem to be so much money around these days. I think that the money should only be spent on those that deserve it, not the people who don't seem to be interested in their health – you know, the ones who eat the wrong food, don't exercise, smoke and ignore any medical advice to change their habits.

Having read the personal stories of Sam and Charmaine you will have built up a mental picture of the two story tellers.

- What has informed this picture?
- Do you feel that the story tellers had been influenced by friends, peers, family or the media?
- What impact have educational experiences had on Sam and Charmaine?
- Are your feelings about the two people influenced by their gender?
- In order to understand the stories did you draw on your own personal experiences, e.g. as carers, workers, members of a family?
- How might you respond to some of their statements?

Think back to the dialogue between Charlie and Andy in Chapter 2. Reflect on the mental picture you have of them. Your value base will affect any response. There are a number of issues here around caring and gender, the deserving and undeserving, the right to intervene in family life and whether personal opinions can affect professional judgements. Take a few minutes before reading on to think about your own personal life and work experiences. What has made you the person you are?

As we said at the start of this chapter, in order for us to engage in the moral and ethical activity that is social care practice the starting point has to be locating ourselves. Otherwise workers and carers will be tossed about among the multitude of dilemmas which exist in practice. In order for us to be able to work effectively it is important that we make decisions which reflect an anti-oppressive perspective rather than being pulled by the dominant currents into oppressive practice.

Values are the codes by which we operate within this social world. They are the moral principles that guide and control our actions. Three types of values can be identified:

- *Ultimate values* are abstract values, such as justice and freedom.
- *Intermediate values* are more explicit to the desired end state but are open to debate, such as the right to an abortion on demand or the right to punish one's child in a certain way.
- *Instrumental values* are modes of conduct, such as confidentiality and self-determination.

Values, then, can be expressed at various levels – from the general level of ideas to the concrete reality of action. Values are not the same as facts, needs, rights or ideologies but they may often be confused. Values are used to reflect what is preferred, whereas facts tell us what actually exists. Rights are legitimate expectations. Ideologies are belief systems containing societal values. In summary, values can be seen as:

- guides to behaviour;
- growing out of personal experiences;
- modified as experiences accumulate;
- evolving in nature (Raths *et al.* 1966).

Values operate within the political, social and economic context. These conditions place conflicting demands on individuals and thus value conflicts will inevitably develop as we are exposed to varying values. This is not to say that we are like puppets with no control over our own actions. Social values direct our action, but we have a part to play in the social drama of life. That is, we incorporate societal values, internally validate them and then, after making them our own, use them to guide our actions.

In locating ourselves and our value base it is important that we engage in what Timms (1983) would identify as *'value talk'*. Ten years ago he stated that 'value talk' was under-developed. His explanation of this was that there was an acceptance of what values meant in social care practice. We would suggest that any attempt to talk about social work values must take into account the confusion that exists between values, beliefs and attitudes. There are those who believe that a definitive list of values exists in social care practice. We would argue, however, that values are not 'empty vessels' but are socially constructed and therefore open to change. Therefore it is impossible to have a definitive list. It is, however, possible to hold on to a set of values that personally informs our practice. What is important is the need to be explicit and prepared to adhere to a coherent framework. This framework incorporates ideas about equality and justice, takes account of positive elements of 'traditional' values (Biestek 1961) and is interrogated by present-day ideas about empowerment (Solomon 1976; Gutierrez 1990; Rees 1991).

Final thoughts

It has been noted by Jordan *et al.* (1993: 7) that there is a

> tension between traditional (liberally generated) professional values, such as rights to individual privacy, confidentiality and choice, and a radical (Marxist) agenda in relation to anti-discriminatory and anti-oppressive policies and practices which must be addressed.

We believe that it is important to interrogate rigorously liberally generated values by using principles, such as empowerment and partnership, that inform anti-oppressive practice. From this inquiry will be formulated the basis of a practice that takes account of the power differentials that exist within society and that if not tackled, enable the status quo to remain.

Activities

Activity 1

Within language are embedded the values, beliefs and ideas which reflect the social, economic and political context in which social work is practised (see Rojek *et al.* 1988). Language can be used to illustrate the power inequalities that exist between individuals and the value judgements which can be made about situations in which people find themselves. With this in mind please read the following poem.

Tomorrow I am going to re-write the English language

Tomorrow I am going to re-write the English language.
I will discard all those striving ambullist metaphors
Of power and success
And construct images to describe my strength.
My new, different strength.
Then I won't have to feel dependent
Because I can't Stand On My Own Two Feet
And I will refuse to feel a failure
Because I didn't Stay One Step Ahead.
I won't feel inadequate
When I don't Stand Up For Myself
Or illogical because I cannot
Just Take It One Step At a Time.

I will make them understand that it is a very male way
To describe the world
All this Walking Tall
And Making Great Strides.

Yes, tomorrow I am going to re-write the English language,
Creating the world in my own image.
Mine will be a gentler, more womanly way
To describe my progress.
I will wheel, cover and encircle

Somehow I will learn to say it all.

(Lois Keith, in Morris 1989)

This poem challenges our assumptions of able-bodiedness and illustrates the way in which our everyday language takes so much for granted. It makes disabled people invisible. Think about what value judgements are portrayed in other poems that you know. Now think about how legislation might reinforce assumptions. Let us look at the legislation around disability. A similar theme of invisibility can be traced.

It was the intention of the Disabled Persons Act 1986 to provide disabled people with a voice, protect their interests and meet their needs – in short it was aimed to minimize their marginalized position. Sections 1 and 2 of the Act provided for the appointment of a representative or advocate to act on behalf of a disabled person in connection with the provision of services. Section 3 requires local authorities to listen to any representations by or on behalf of the person with a disability, and to provide a written statement of needs and proposals to meet them. None of these sections have been implemented. The message behind the decision not to implement these sections is 'you are invisible' – if you are invisible you have no rights, you have no status, you are oppressed.

It is of course easy to criticize the fact that legislation has not been implemented, and to analyse why this might be so. From our perspective, however, we would argue that the fact that it has been discussed and written down is a starting point, and provides a lever to promote future change. It also does not mean that good practice should not prevail: Sections 1 to 3 can, and should, provide guidelines to good practice in promoting anti-oppressive practice in work with people who are disabled.

Now think of ways, using legislation, in which you can enable people with disabilities to become visible.

Activity 2

Below are a number of statements which you may well have heard or used at some time. When you are reading them please try to identify:

- the social and ethical values on which the statements might be based;
- possible hidden assumptions, which are oppressive in effect, behind these statements;
- how you would use the legislation to support your reply.

1 'I favour equal rights for the disabled – I've made several suggestions of ways we can help them.'
2 'The council is spending a lot on minority cultures – what about our needs?'
3 'I personally have no say in this institution's policies, sexist, disabilist, elitist or otherwise.'
4 'I treat all people the same – in our organization we make no difference between people.'

Although these appear to be quite simple statements they convey complex issues, which, depending on your value base, can be answered in a number of ways.

Activity 3

An understanding of popular language and the values it implies can be obtained by scrutinizing media reporting. Read the following newspaper story.

Home alone at Christmas
In the early hours of Christmas Eve 1993 three small girls were taken into care. They were sisters aged between ten months and ten years. Their mother was 25. The family lived together in a council house. The house was in a poor state of repair, it was dirty, carpets were covered with cat and dog faeces, half eaten food littered the front room. The cooker in the kitchen was encased in grease, the fetid air made it difficult for police and social workers to breathe without feeling as though they were going to be physically sick. The children were found alone when police and social workers called.

The social worker's story
This is not a 'home alone' case. The mother was with her children. Concern was about neglect – neglect linked to poverty. The poverty was not caused by any extravagant lifestyle but by an insensitive benefits system. This case is one of many that this office deals with. What should be of concern is that this is a case we are aware of. There are many others that are not brought to our attention.

But what we are sure of is that this case highlights the nature of deprivation, poverty and inequality that some families experience.

The mother's story
It hurts to see your story splashed all over the newspaper, particularly when all the facts are wrong. I have had social workers calling round all the time, checking on my children and helping me with the housing and the social. Things were going all right for a time until my fella, Ronnie, walked out on me and the kids. That was in August. I was upset by this but you have to get on with your life, so I carried on best I could.

I met Peter in November and that's when things really got difficult. Ronnie saw me and Peter together and started getting funny with me. He didn't want to know before, but because I was with someone else he felt he owned me. Anyway, Ronnie called round saying he wanted to see the children, but he called at eight, nine or ten o'clock at night sometimes and I would say no, he couldn't, because they were in bed. There would be an argument. Peter would say something, Ronnie would tell him to 'shut it', 'cos he wasn't the girls' father. The baby would wake up and that would be the end of my night with Peter.

Just before Christmas, Ronnie wanted the children to spend Christmas with him. I said no and a row started. Ronnie left, saying he was going to get the social workers and the police on to me. He said that I was too busy with Peter to mind the children properly. Social workers and police have called out a few times now – he tells them a pack of lies, but it's their job, they have to check the children are OK. Ronnie has applied for an order to see them. I didn't mind him seeing the children – it's the time. You can't come round at night to see a baby can you?

Anyway, on Christmas Eve morning, Ronnie called round, said he had presents for the children out in the car. So I let them go out to get their presents. I was standing by the door. Next thing, Ronnie drives off with the children. So I called the police, told them what had happened. I went out to look for them. When I got back, the police were at the house. Ronnie had just gone round the block. He had come back and got in the house, left the children and then called the police on me. When I got in, the police asked why I had left the children on their own. They said that they were taking them into care and that social workers had found somewhere for them. I saw red then, and grabbed my kids. I was crying and screaming and so were they. When the social workers came I just ran out of the house. I couldn't take any more. Now my girls are in care.

The social services director's story
I cannot comment on a specific case but this case has to be seen in a wider context of poverty and deprivation. The benefits system has failed this family. People like this mother find it difficult to manage on the limited income they get from the state. Christmas is a financially difficult time, particularly when you have children. But these cases don't just come to light at Christmas. We see cases like this every day of every week. People find it hard to cope, they are not parents who do not care. They care very much. But they do not have the financial resources to care properly for their children. They know this, and the stress of

knowing, of being unable to do something, is very great and sometimes people break.

1 What basic values are being expressed through the media and the stories of the people involved?
2 What impact does the mother's story have on you?
3 What impact do you think the media has had on the mother?
4 What are the arguments put forward by the media to the public by their presentation of her story?
5 How would your own value base affect your response at a practical, policy and legislative level?
6 You are one of the people involved in the mother's life (you could for example be the babysitter, personal friend, health visitor, or school nurse). What is your story? Once you have written it write an imaginary letter to the paper that printed the article.

This exercise is based on an article printed in the *Guardian*, 19 January 1994.

4   EMPOWERMENT

Warning

When I am an old woman I shall wear purple
With a red hat which doesn't go, and doesn't suit me,
And I shall spend my pension on brandy and summer gloves
And satin sandals, and say we've no money for butter.
I shall sit down on the pavement when I'm tired
And gobble up samples in shops and press alarm bells
And run my stick along public railings
And make up for the sobriety of my youth.
I shall go out in my slippers in the rain
And pick the flowers in other people's gardens
And learn to spit.

You can wear terrible shirts and grow more fat
And eat three pounds of sausages at a go
Or only eat bread and pickle for a week
And hoard pens and pencils and beer mats and things in boxes.
But now we must have clothes that keep us dry
And pay our rent and not swear in the street
And set a good example for the children.
We will have friends to dinner and read the papers.
But maybe I ought to practise a little now?
So people who know me are not too shocked and surprised
When suddenly I am old and start to wear purple.

(Jenny Joseph 1985)

Personal social services have a huge resource in terms of
hard working and skilled staff who have a vision of greater
empowerment for users and carers. Indeed, what we have seen
and heard is deeply moving. It shows workers creating 'islands' of
empowerment over matters in which they have influence, in the

deep and turbulent sea of social disempowerment through
poverty, racism, unemployment and homelessness.
(Stevenson and Parsloe 1993: 13)

Introduction

If we start from an understanding that 'social work is an intellectual activity
that has practical application' (Anderson 1993) then we have a responsibility
to analyse critically the concepts that we use in our day-to-day working with
service users or those we are caring for and in our communication (direct
and indirect) with our colleagues. We will begin by asking you to reflect on
what empowerment means to you. We will then briefly review the more
recent development of the notion of empowerment before considering some
definitions. This provides the backdrop against which we develop our own
model of empowerment. In Chapter 1 we saw that the central element in
thinking about oppression is that all relationships are characterized by a
power dimension. So empowerment practice incorporates this issue and,
informed by duality theory, has a view of society where people do not just
have individual relationships but are also part of wider structures. There are
unequal balances of power within and between these relationships and so
empowerment is about understanding and trying to balance them. The model
we develop explains the process of empowerment, which incorporates the
relationships between individuals and the society in which we live.

The term *empowerment* is a concept that has had a considerable impact
upon the nature of social care practice. It was the 'buzz word' of the late
1980s (Adams 1990) and it has become more popular in the 1990s as a term
used to reflect the nature of social care or 'to describe a movement towards
greater equality of the parties who relate to each other in community care'
(Stevenson and Parsloe 1993: 6). Stevenson and Parsloe go on to point out
that, although the term is not often used in government guidance, the
notion of empowerment does underpin recent legislation; for instance, 'it is
placed centre-stage in the influential Managers and Practitioners Guide to
Care Management and Assessment' (Stevenson and Parsloe 1993: 9), which
states that 'the rationale for this reorganisation is the empowerment of users
and carers' (DoH 1991b; quoted in Stevenson and Parsloe 1993: 9).

With the establishment of the notion of empowerment has also come a
critique of its meaning. So what does the term really mean? Is it just a word
that has become fashionable for use by professionals and politicians? Is it
used as a synonym for enabling? Does it, as Ward and Mullender (1991)
suggest, lack specificity and gloss over significant difference? Or, as Croft and
Beresford (1989) argue, is it a much abused and devalued word?

What does the term 'empowerment' mean to you? You may find it helpful
to jot down a few ideas that come to mind. Can you think of a time when
you have felt empowered? Describe the situation. Who was involved? How
did you feel? How did you respond? We all have different experiences of

being empowered which lead us to an understanding of what empowerment means to us. Having done this exercise you will have come up with at least some of the following ideas about empowerment:

- gaining more control over your own life;
- being aware of and using your personal resources;
- overcoming obstacles to meeting your needs and aspirations;
- having your voice heard in decision making;
- being able to challenge inequality and oppression in your life (adapted from Kirton and Virdee 1992).

This is not an exhaustive list. You may wish to add to it.

To summarize, to empower one has to be able to hold on to and defend one's value perspective, and have some critical awareness of the interaction that takes place between individuals. The essence of empowerment can be simply stated: it is about not making assumptions and asking the question why. Critical analysis is the forerunner of empowerment.

Development of the concept of empowerment

Legislation in the past 20 years has enhanced the statutory powers available to workers in the social care field. There is the potential, therefore, for users to feel further disempowered by the use of such legislation. We have already noted that the notion of empowerment in social care is an expected element of practice in both official and professional arenas (Stevenson and Parsloe 1993). But there are a number of crucial questions which writers such as Croft and Beresford (1989) have asked. Can people really have more say in social services? Is it a practical possibility? How do we manage the ethical dilemmas that empowerment practice poses?

Jordan (1990) argues that service users and practitioners need to meet together as fellow citizens, to reason together about the ethical dilemmas they face. This, he suggests, means meeting together in the context of relations within their society, i.e. laws, conventions and values, and also within a wider context of human relations. Stevenson and Parsloe (1993: 15) also recognize the dilemmas facing practitioners in decision making:

> Ethical dilemmas . . . arise in the application of the ideal. Our conversation with social workers suggested a minefield of ethical issues and dilemmas, too little discussed, rumbling on in the minds and feelings of practitioners.

Such dilemmas include concerns about 'risk', the question of whether it is possible to work in true partnership and how far participation of users is merely tokenism.

Broadly one finds empowerment publicly associated with two competing concepts. One is the New Right's welfare consumerism and the other is the user movement. Privately the word is used by individuals so that they can be seen to be progressive and credible (Croft and Beresford 1989). The concept of empowerment, then, needs to be clearly defined, with the aim of using it as a tool for change. Hence it is important that it is intellectually interrogated.

In tracing the historical development of the term empowerment, Barbara Bryant Solomon's work *Black Empowerment* provides us with a useful starting point. Solomon (1976: 12) refers to empowerment

> as a process whereby persons who belong to a stigmatized social category throughout their lives can be assisted to develop and increase skills in the exercise of interpersonal influence and the performance of valued social roles.

The major thesis of her book is that individuals and groups in black communities have been subjected to negative valuations from the larger society to such an extent that powerlessness in the group is pervasive and crippling. Although Solomon talks specifically about black communities in the United States of America, her work has major relevance to other negatively valued groups in this society. Solomon argues that empowerment is about engaging service users in the problem solving process. This process serves to counteract the oppressions that shape and inform the lives of those who do not have access, or have limited access, to the power structures of society.

How can we engage people in the problem solving process? One of the ways of doing this is by enabling people to talk about their experiences of oppression. By documenting the experiences of black women, black female writers (Lorde 1984; hooks 1989; Hill-Collins 1990) have shown that if women are to take control of their lives they need to articulate and share their experiences of oppression. By making visible their personal experiences they begin to value themselves – which of itself is empowering. Once empowered they are able to start the process of rejecting the system which perpetuates their oppression. Taking this point into consideration we must therefore look at the structure and process of service delivery systems that have the greatest potential for facilitating empowerment of service users, i.e. involving them in the problem solving process. Our services must be sensitive – a sensitivity that can only be brought about by practitioners listening to and taking account of people's experiences. As Solomon (1976: 29) points out, 'The success or failure of empowerment is directly related to the degree to which [the] service delivery system itself is an obstacle course or an opportunity system.'

Definitions

How do we use the law, within our services, as an opportunity system? A study of the literature about empowerment practice indicates that it is a process (Rappaport 1985; Rees 1991; Phillipson 1992; Stevenson and Parsloe 1993). That process is dynamic. However, not only is it a process, it is also a goal (Swift and Levin 1987) or a product (Holdsworth 1991) – the 'end state'. But what is the process? The experiences of black women provide us with a handle on the process of empowerment. Solomon (1976: 19), discussing social work with black people, states that empowerment is the process whereby the social worker engages in a set of activities with the client or client system that aim to reduce the powerlessness that has been created by negative valuations based on membership in a stigmatized group.

Gutierrez (1990: 149), in identifying a set of principles of empowering practice for 'women of color', sees it as 'a process of increasing personal, interpersonal, or political power so that individuals can take action to improve their life situations'. Rappaport (1984: 3) also identifies and links the personal and political aspects of empowerment, describing it as a way that 'people, organisations and communities gain mastery over their own lives'. For Rappaport (1987: 121) it 'conveys both a psychological sense of personal control or influence and a concern with actual social influence, political power, and legal rights'. DuBois and Krogsrud Miley (1992: 42) define empowerment as

a process of releasing the potential and strengths of social systems and discovering and creating resources and opportunities for promoting adaptive social functioning in the client system's resolution of problems, issues and needs.

They clearly see the levels of power as interrelated.

Empowerment as a concept, however, becomes meaningful when we relate it to power and oppression:

empowerment, if connected with a notion of oppression . . . can become a distinctive underpinning for practice, and one which does not become colonised or domesticated in the service of the status quo.

(Mullender and Ward 1991: 22)

Empowerment as a process

During the depression years of the 1930s, cookery classes were organised for women in poor communities in an attempt to help them to provide nutritious meals for their families despite their low incomes. One particular evening a group of women were being taught how to make cod's head soup – a cheap and nourishing dish. At the end of the lesson the women were asked if they had any questions. 'Just one', said a member of the group, 'whilst we're eating the cod's head soup, who's eating the cod?'

(Popay and Dhooge 1989: 140)

The first stage of empowerment is about making the links between our personal position and structural inequalities. For the woman in the cookery class the question indicated the start of a process of awareness about her position. This position was not about knowing that she was poor, i.e. her personal position, but was about making the links between the personal and the structural, i.e. access to power and resources. Empowerment can be seen in terms of process and goal (Swift and Levin 1987; Stevenson and Parsloe

1993). It is about replacing powerlessness with 'some sense of power' so that 'confusion can give way to a feeling of coherence' (Rees 1991: 21). Health and social care practitioners do not instantly *give* people power; rather, as indicated by Barbara Solomon, they aim to help reduce the powerlessness that individuals and groups experience.

An empowerment perspective which assumes that issues of power and powerlessness are integral to the experience of the service user enables us to move away from pathologizing individuals to increasing personal, interpersonal or political power so that individuals can take action to improve their life situations. Within the existing models of social care practice there is a focus on the individual – problems are individualized (blame the victim syndrome). Interventions often focus on assisting individuals to cope with or accept a difficult situation rather than changing the situation on a structural level.

At a micro-level empowerment is described as the development of a personal feeling of increased power or control without an actual change in structural arrangements. Empowerment on a macro-level is seen as a process of increasing collective political power. A third level of empowerment relates to the interface of these two approaches: individual empowerment can contribute to group empowerment and, in turn, the increase in a group's power can enhance the functioning of its individual members.

If empowerment practice is to be effective it is essential to understand the process which leads from feeling powerless to powerful. This process is a process of change – which is what anti-oppressive practice is about. The process will go through a number of stages and occur at a number of levels. Rappaport (1984) describes the process as being multifaceted and multidimensional. Rees (1991), in outlining a scheme for practice based on the work of Friere (1972), Rose and Black (1985) and Rosenfeld (1989), talks about the mutuality of interaction between the stages, and develops a scheme for practice that proceeds through a number of stages, which he describes as an 'educational device' rather than a mechanical scheme to be rigidly followed.

Other writers also discuss empowerment practice taking place on different levels. Thompson (1993) develops a model which identifies empowerment taking place at the personal, cultural and institutional levels. Hasenfield (1987: 479) also identifies three levels, the *worker–client* level, which is involved with 'improving the client's power resources', the *organizational* level, which is aimed 'generally at harnessing the agency's power advantages to increasingly serve the needs of the client', and the *policy* level, which ensures that 'the formulation and enactment of policy decisions are influenced by those directly affected by them'. Troyna and Hatcher (1992), in their model for analysing racist incidents in schools, move through eight levels from the interactional to the structural. However, these can be broadly grouped into three levels which, like the others, can equate with the perspective put forward by Rappaport (1985) that a person can take control of her or his own life at the level of feelings, the level of ideas and the level of being able to make a difference to the world around him or her, or the level of activity.

The model we have developed in trying to understand the process of empowerment is therefore informed by the work of a number of writers. It is informed by 'a belief that power is not a scarce commodity but rather one that can be generated in the process of empowerment' (Gutierrez 1990: 150).

The first level is the *level of feeling*. This level is very much concerned with the personal experiences of the person who is feeling powerless. A number of elements can be identified at this level based on these experiences.

It is impossible to begin change without first being able to locate oneself. Rees (1991: 86) points out that 'the processes of empowerment may cover the story of a lifetime'. He talks about the 'promise of biography', which he explains as 'the telling of a story with a view to participating in a different way in future events' (Rees 1991: 21). From the telling of the story, Rees explains, the one who is being listened to will become more confident in the knowledge that she or he is being taken seriously. This confidence is empowering. Certain *themes* will also emerge, so that links can be made between personal and social issues. This notion is based on the work of Freire, who, by involving people oppressed by poverty in critical *dialogue*, enabled them to engage in praxis – analysing social situations and acting on that analysis. Hill-Collins (1990) points out that the process of self-conscious thought is an essential element of the empowerment process, with personal experience thus being a central element. In their model for analysing racist incidents Troyna and Hatcher (1992) begin with three stages, which all concentrate on the 'feelings' level. The first is *interactional*, concentrating on the actual incident: what was done, what was said. The next is *contextual*: the immediate history of the racist incident. The third is *biographical*: the factors and characteristics specific to the individuals involved in the incident. It is this level which Hill-Collins would call the process of self-conscious struggle.

We can see this summarized in the centre of Figure 4.1, where the level of feelings is focused on personal biography. This is the core of the empowerment process.

The second level is the *level of ideas*, which according to Rappaport (1985) is about self-worth. It is about increasing self-efficacy, i.e. a belief in the ability 'to produce and regulate events in one's life' (Bandura 1982: 122). Gutierrez explains that although this term has not been used in much empowerment literature a similar phenomenon is described by most authors and involves such concepts as strengthening ego functioning, developing a sense of personal power or strength, developing a sense of control, developing client initiative or increasing the client's ability to act. This continuing process of self-conscious struggle leads to a changed consciousness – self-knowledge, self-actualization, self-definition. This in itself will lead to increased self-respect as people learn to evaluate their self-image and thus gain knowledge about themselves (Rees 1991).

At this level, then, people are able to reduce self-blame – Gutierrez explains that powerlessness leads to depression and immobilization. Raised consciousness and an understanding that we are not responsible for the negative situation enables us to 'shift focus'. We then move from feeling defective or deficient to feeling more capable of changing the situation. We can do this because we are able to attribute problems to existing power structures in society. Much of the process at this level has connections with humanist and existential models and 'emphasises values of self knowledge

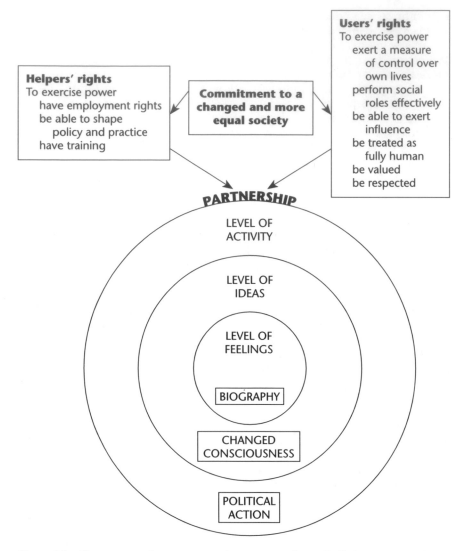

Figure 4.1   The process of empowerment: a process of growth that may occur at any time. Change at any one level will affect change at other levels.

and self control which also accept that clients have rational cognitive control of their lives' (Payne 1991: 227). Troyna and Hatcher identify three stages within the level of ideas in relation to young people in school: the *subcultural*, the *institutional* and the *cultural*. At the institutional stage are what they call the 'ideologies, procedural norms and practices which are promoted, sanctioned and diffused by the school', while at the cultural level they also refer to experiences of young people in terms of their 'lived experience and

common-sense understanding', both locally, particularly through family networks, and within the community generally.

Developing self-knowledge and thus, at the level of ideas, a sense of personal power, enables people to develop new language. Rees (1991) sees language not merely as a device for communicating but also as 'a means of
creating social relationships and realising the self involved in those relationships' (Rees 1991: 95). As connections are made between one's own story
or personal biography and the biographies of other people, the insight thus
gained will be indicated by new words which form a language that expresses
power, e.g. 'I want to make my own choices', 'I know my rights', 'I'm in
control'.

The level of ideas is represented in the second band of Figure 4.1, which
identifies the elements that at this level must inevitably lead to a changed
consciousness.

The level of *action* is about moving from the personal to the political. For
Hasenfield (1987: 479; quoted in Holdsworth 1991: 11) it is about ensuring
that 'the formulation and enactment of policy decisions are influenced by
those directly affected by them'. One of the five skills identified by Solomon
as necessary for empowerment practice is the need to facilitate organizational change, which she sees as an agency related form of intervention in
both policy and practice. This is made possible through the development of
raised consciousness and the subsequent awareness of the possibility of
political and social action. Hill-Collins (1990) states that the process of political
action is not an end in itself for any one particular group. It is about an
ability to work with others to change social institutions. However, it is assisted through the development of group consciousness, which involves the
development of an awareness of how political structures affect both individual
and group experiences (Gutierrez 1990). At this level there is a very real
danger that people feel doubt about the action they have been taking. This
is an inevitable part of the process of growing stronger and may be evidenced in a desire for the familiar. It is often far easier to return to a difficult
but familiar situation than it is to fight on. It is at this point, therefore, that
the person will need the appropriate support if she or he is to resist returning
to the former state of powerlessness (Rees 1991). The objectives of empowerment at this level may be about changing legislation or policies, but can
equally be about the small changes that may affect the life of one individual,
which in Rappaport's (1985) terms is about making a difference in the world
around us.

Although these levels have been described in an order, the empowerment
process does not occur in an ordered step-by-step way. It is an ongoing
process with shifting goals. The changes can often occur at the same time at
various levels and so enhance one another. As Gutierrez notes, researchers who
have studied the process suggest that one does not 'achieve empowerment';
it is a continual process of growth and change which can occur throughout
one's lifetime (Friere 1972; Kieffer 1984).

The model we have developed provides a framework to cover both the
micro and the macro, i.e. the personal and the political (Phillipson 1992).
In the diagrammatic representation of the model (Figure 4.1) the circles

represent the process of empowerment at the different levels. This can only successfully operate when all those involved in the process are working in partnership with a joint commitment to a changed and more equal society.

The level of activity surrounds the whole of the empowerment process because it is the all-encompassing element of the process, taking in both the personal and the structural and involving change through political action. The circular diagram identifies how the process is one which is interlinked but also occurs at any or all of the levels at any one time. The process is circular. Change at the level of feelings will affect the level of ideas as self-awareness develops. This in turn can enable a mobilization of resources at the level of action. This then affects one's biography at the level of feelings, as inevitably change has occurred. And so the process goes on.

It may well be, however, that the process begins at the level of action, which will lead to a changed consciousness and again affect the personal biography. Essentially change occurring at one level must effect change at other levels. The relationship between health and welfare practitioners or carers and the person they are working with is crucial, however, to enable the process to take place.

To summarize, the process of empowerment occurs on individual, inter-personal and institutional levels. Thus an individual is able to develop a sense of personal power, an ability to affect others and an ability to work with others to change social institutions. The approach then sees change as a move from the personal to the political.

Principles and assumptions of empowerment

DuBois and Krogsrud Miley (1992) list a number of guiding principles and assumptions underlying the process of empowerment* which have been described by various authors (Solomon 1976; Rappaport 1981, 1984; Pinder-hughes 1983; Swift 1984; Swift and Levin 1987; Weick *et al.* 1989).

- Empowerment is a collaborative process, with the client and the practitioner working together as partners.
- The empowering process views the client systems as competent and capable, given access to resources and opportunities.
- Clients must first perceive themselves as causal agents, able to effect change.
- Competence is acquired or refined through life experiences, particularly experience affirming efficacy, rather than from circumstances where one is told what to do.
- Solutions, evolving from the particular situation, are necessarily diverse and emphasize 'complexities of multiple contributory factors in any problem situation' (Solomon 1976: 27).
- Informal social networks are a significant source of support for mediating stress and increasing one's competence and sense of control.

---

* From Brenda DuBois and Karla Krogsrud Miley, *Social Work: An Empowering Profession.* Copyright © 1992 by Allyn and Bacon. Reprinted by permission.

- People must participate in their own empowerment; goals, means and outcomes must be self-defined.
- Level of awareness is a key issue in empowerment; 'knowledge mobilises action for change' (Swift and Levin 1987: 81).
- Empowerment involves access to resources and the capacity to use those resources in an effective way.
- The empowering process is dynamic, synergistic, ever changing and evolutionary; problems always have multiple solutions.
- Empowerment is achieved through the parallel structures of personal and socio-economic development.

These principles should underpin our practice if it is to be truly empowering.

Making the connections

In trying to understand what empowerment really means we first need to review our discussions about oppression in Part I of the book. Oppression is a complex term – it is not one-dimensional but multi-faceted and it is easy to be overwhelmed by the sheer scale of the problem. A critical model is needed, therefore, to see what is going on. As with 'empowerment', the word 'oppression' can often be used without an understanding of what it means, as discussed in Chapter 1. Oppression itself is a powerful force. On a personal level it can lead to demoralization and lack of self-esteem, while at a structural level it can lead to denial of rights.

For us oppression is best understood if it is seen as a system of *colliding explosive forces*, which, if they collide randomly, are more likely to be oppressive. If channelled and controlled, however, they can open up new opportunities. A controlled explosion is more likely to have a positive outcome than one over which there is no control. The generation of power within that explosive situation can be harnessed to be a positive energizing force, rather than one that is left to dissipate and have negative consequences. Therefore, in our practice and use of legislation, we must acknowledge all these competing forces. We must get them to work together and become more stable, so that the outcome is positive.

To illustrate the above point let us briefly analyse the case of *R* v *Devon County Council ex parte L* [1991] 2 FLR 541. We have used this case, which can be seen to be controversial, because:

- it is a documented case, which actually happened;
- it presents a number of ethical and moral dilemmas;
- it enables us to consider issues about men who abuse children;
- it enables us to consider issues about the power of adults over children;
- it provides the opportunity to consider the principles of empowerment in a difficult situation;
- in working with offenders practitioners will often find themselves working in oppressive situations, and it is important not to intensify this position for the offender or alleged offender.

The answers we provide are hypothetical, based on the facts made available to us.

The facts

The case concerns an alleged child sexual abuser, Mr L. In 1986 he moved into the home of a Mrs B and shortly afterwards they began to live together as man and wife. However, he moved out in August 1987. Mrs B had two children. In December 1987 the headmistress of the school of the elder child (born 1982) contacted social services because of concern about her disturbing behaviour. Mrs B's daughter was examined by a consultant paediatrician and stated in the presence of the doctor and a social worker that Mr L had been touching her in an inappropriate manner. Some inflammation of the vagina was found but no bruising or contusions. The paediatrician took the view that although there was no physical evidence of abuse the examination findings were consistent with manipulation of her genital area.

Following a visit by representatives of the NSPCC and a female police constable a report was written which indicated that Mr L had sexually assaulted Mrs B's daughter. He was arrested and interviewed on the same day and denied the allegations. No criminal proceedings were ever instituted against Mr L.

In June 1988, the applicant started to live with Mrs G. She became pregnant by Mr L and later gave birth to his child. Three incidents occurred between June 1988 and September 1990. On each occasion Mr L started to live with women who were subsequently advised by social workers that if he remained in the household a case conference would have to be held to discuss possible registration of the children who lived there. In the first two cases Mr L moved out following a request to leave by the women concerned. In the third case he did not leave immediately and there were several visits by social workers as well as some correspondence. On one occasion a letter to one of the women suggested that the local authority might have to consider care proceedings in the case of her granddaughter.

The issues

1 At no time was Mr L's name on a list of abusers or child abuse register.
2 Social work intervention was not as a result of any case conference decision.
3 Four social workers believed that they were carrying out their duties.
4 None of the social workers had interviewed Mr L but they knew that he had been interviewed by police – although no police action had been taken.
5 Each believed the allegations made by the child.
6 Mr L was illiterate and so had a different understanding of the allegations.

It was stated by Hayes (1992) that 'The social work practice in the Devon case is open to criticism on three main counts. It was high handed, it was partly ineffectual and it was unfair.' Let us consider these questions from an anti-oppressive perspective. It could be argued that if the practitioners had been informed by an empowerment perspective this case might never have been brought before the court.

Q: What was the evidence that this action was high handed?

A: The social workers made no real attempt to work in partnership with the various women that Mr L had been involved with: they could have involved the women in plans about protecting their children; they could have explained clearly the options available rather than taking a coercive approach.

Q: Why was it partly ineffectual?

A: Two of the women managed to conceal the fact that Mr L had at some stage returned to the household. Therefore contact with the children thought to be at risk was not prevented.

Q: Why was it unfair?

A: First, Mr L was not given an opportunity to be heard. Secondly, he was not given the opportunity to be a part of the assessment of risk and thus to indicate how he might no longer pose a threat to the children concerned in order to allay the fears of the authorities.

Therefore a just and comprehensive assessment for preventing Mr L from living in households with children did not take place.

Analysis

The above case can be analysed by using the colliding forces framework.

Colliding forces

It is important to take account of the different power relationships that exist. In this case there were a number of competing interests. They are as follows:

- between different professionals;
- between professionals and Mr L;
- between professionals and the women;
- between professionals and the children;
- between Mr L and each of the three women;
- between Mr L and the various children involved (i.e. from the child who had originally made the allegations, his child by Mrs G and the children of the other families).

It is important also to take account of gender, race, age, class, disability and other social divisions which play a part in determining the power relationships in this situation. This also adds to the miscommunication, which may then become explosive. From the evidence, the starting point for practitioners was that the child was at risk. That ignited the situation. Mr L experienced a number of feelings, one of which was a sense of powerlessness, and therefore sought the assistance of a solicitor, which brings a new element into the equation.

Channelling the power

If we view the situation from Mr L's perspective for a moment, he was insufficiently involved in the local authority's decision making process. That process led to a number of his personal family relationships being broken up and to him losing contact with his own child. If work had been in partnership with Mr L he would have been given the opportunity to understand what risk was presented and to work jointly towards change in order to minimize that risk. In that work there would be some recognition of whether it was possible for him to live within a household with children. It would also be good practice to have two workers involved in the case in order to minimize the conflict of roles. This would in fact be a more effective way of working – and legislation does allow for working in partnership.

Obviously there is a conflict of interests if only one worker is involved: how easy would it be to keep the interests of the child paramount if you were also working with the alleged 'abuser'? By entering into dialogue with Mr L you are empowering him by engaging him in the process. This then channels the negative energy of Mr L, which could be seen in his use of the law (actively seeking the help of a solicitor to take his case to court). It also channels the power of the social workers into opening up new opportunities which work more effectively and are less likely to violate anyone's rights.

Harnessing the power

Mr L could continue in the same pattern because he is disempowered by the process and his treatment by the professionals involved. He also could seek further recourse to the law and appeal to the Court of Human Rights under Article 8, on the grounds that he was insufficiently involved in the local authority's decision making process. That process led to a number of his personal family relationships being broken up and to him losing contact with his child. Thus, Hayes (1992) points out, failure to afford Mr L proper procedural safeguards when intervening to this degree in his family life put Devon County Council in breach of Article 8.

If the power was harnessed appropriately the positive force that might be generated within him might help him to understand the very real concerns of the statutory agencies. He would then be able to work with them in order to minimize the risk that he is seen to pose to the children.

Anti-oppressive practice is about ensuring that people are not oppressed because of the protective nature of our role. It is difficult to think about anti-oppressive practice when working with someone whom we believe may well have abused his own power (as a male adult). So the practice is about helping that person to understand why his action has been seen as an abuse of power. The purpose of anti-oppressive practice in situations like this is summed up by Malcolm Payne (1994: 6): 'We should stop the perpetrator of sexual or domestic violence from damaging others. At the same time we should aim to free them from the social and personal bonds which lead to their behaviour.'

Final thoughts

The model of empowerment we have developed is one which we use in our practice. Through our personal experiences we have discovered the importance of biography. As we have moved through the process of looking at ourselves and using those experiences to inform our action we have found that action in turn has been woven into our biography. This has then had an impact on our level of ideas, feelings and activity. And so the process goes on as we grow and develop. The process is an 'evolving process which has no end point, which may explain the reluctance and fear with which it is sometimes regarded' (Stevenson and Parsloe 1993: 10).

Activity

Read the following case scenario.

B v B (Grandparents: Residence Order) Re

An application made for a residence order in respect of a girl aged 11 by her maternal grandmother and supported by her mother was refused by the justices on the grounds that the court should not make an order unless doing so would be better than making no order at all (Section 1(5)). Since the girl had lived with the grandmother for all but the first six weeks of her life and it had been agreed by the mother and grandmother, the justices found there was no risk of the child being taken away from her present home.

Bearing in mind the principles of empowerment that have previously been discussed, do you feel that this was the right decision by the court in terms of empowering the grandmother and her granddaughter?

The grandmother went to appeal. What grounds do you think she might have for an appeal? Think about what might have motivated the grandmother to use the law in this way in the first place, as it is not an easy thing to do. Bear in mind how the granddaughter might feel when she cannot immediately get a response to a request to go on a school trip. Think about the grandmother's situation in a medical emergency. What conclusions do you come to about anti-oppressive practice and the making of an order?

Commentary
This is what actually happened. On appeal an order was made because:

1 The grandmother had found that the education authorities were reluctant to accept her authority in matters where consent was required (e.g. school trips) and had insisted on having the written authority of the mother.
2 There were likely to be situations in the child's life where emergency medical attention was required and where the grandmother's consent was deemed inadequate.
3 There were reasons to believe that the mother's behaviour was sometimes impulsive and that pressures upon her might lead to her removing the child from the grandmother.
4 There was evidence that the child was disturbed by the seeming lack of stability in the arrangements made for her.

In those respects it would be better for the child in this instance if the order were made, particularly as Section 12(2) also provides that the person in whose favour the residence order is made shall have parental responsibility (Hargrove 1992).

Douglas (1992) points out that while his Lordship, Johnson J, might have considered the case somewhat unusual, it remains a fact that there will be reasons for pressing for an order, e.g. to convince dubious housing authorities of one's priority need for accommodation (Yell 1992) or to persuade doctors or education authorities of the standing of a person.

5 PARTNERSHIP

His social worker came to visit,
And went through the work she had begun.
Everything he had asked
Was almost done.
Together they discussed possibilities
of the future – which was to come.
Many options she gave him
Which made it hard to decide which one.
She asked for his permission,
To do the things she wanted to do.
Happily he agreed.
The fact is she asked!

(Chrissie Elms Bennett 1994)

The notion of including service users as participants in decisions about the organization of social care services is not new. The Seebohm Report (1968) mentioned citizen participation in outlining a community based family orientated service. The Barclay Report (1982: 198) suggested 'that personal social services must develop a close working partnership with citizens focusing more clearly on the community and its strength'. Citizens here are partners who should directly participate in agency decision making, while workers are accountable to all those with whom they have a partnership relationship. In this chapter we will explore the concept of partnership, bearing in mind the discussions about empowerment in the previous chapter. We will then consider various partnership approaches and look at how power relationships can be used to promote the rights of users and carers and the problems that can occur.

What do we mean by partnership?

There have been varying developments over the years and the principle of including users has developed, perhaps more noticeably with people with learning disabilities, in the mental health field and in the practice of some residential and day care facilities. Jordan (1990) suggests that the terms associated with these developments are ones like *community social work, participation* and *normalization*, as well as partnership. Nevertheless, as Collins and Stein (1989: 85) point out, it still remains 'a highly problematic concept as well as an undeveloped practice'. While the Children Act 1989, for example, emphasizes the importance of partnership, a National Inspection of Services to Disabled Children in 1993 found that despite evidence of much positive practice, a partnership approach was lacking in a number of significant areas:

- in involving parents on management and planning groups for services;
- in ensuring regular feedback from parents about the quality of services they received;
- in working with parents from different ethnic groups to ensure that services were appropriate and accessible (DoH 1994).

Partnership can mean anything from the most cautious interpretations (as in Barclay) to the most radical (Croft and Beresford 1992, 1993), including what Arnstein (1969) has highlighted as non-participation, varying degrees of tokenism and user power. What links both ends of the spectrum is the notion that service users should be included as far as possible as fellow citizens in the decision making processes which affect their lives. Agencies, professional workers and carers should be enabling users to be full citizens rather than excluding them from decision making processes. Some of the problematic issues around the notion of partnership can often be ignored, such as the relationship between professionalism and participation, social control and democracy, consumerism and elected representation. Cautious interpretations especially emphasize the need to identify and contain those who are defined as dangerous or labelled as disturbed. Dilemmas are then raised around notions of 'risk'.

Problems are also raised by the necessity of working within the effects of existing stereotyping and labelling. For instance, Frost and Stein (1989) argue that state agencies should act in partnership with parents in their child rearing, suggesting that such a model of shared care is offered as a relief service to families under pressure. Thus they see care as a non-stigmatizing service which could be used to assist families and children in facing and working through their problems. Similarly, partnership in day care could provide a more flexible system to meet the needs of black children, single parent families, women and so on. Arguably the Children Act has attempted to do just that. The legislation recognizes the need to provide preventive services for families. Care should only be used as a last resort. Nevertheless, many young people who are accommodated by local authorities consider themselves to be *in care* and stigmatized accordingly. Equally, those families who are in receipt of services in order to help them to look after their children, do not necessarily feel that they are working in partnership with the service providers.

It is important to remember that user groups are invariably marginalized. Leonard (1984) points out that first they can be marginalized within their own environment – seen as a *threat* within their own community. This then forces *isolation* upon them and thus they become labelled as offenders, disabled, elderly, unemployed, etc. These labels come from within the dominant ideologies. In practice this affects how so-called expert professionals view partnership, since service users are often unable to represent themselves in a meaningful way, so that their wishes and feelings will often have to be expressed through the involvement of practitioners (Rojek *et al.* 1988).

In discussing the need for a statement of principles for empowering practice, Stevenson and Parsloe (1993: 39) quote a framework used by Social Work in Partnership, a project involving both children and adults based in two different local authorities. The agreed principles of the project were:

1 Investigations of problems must be with the explicit consent of the potential user(s) and client(s) (in this terminology a client is an involuntary user).
2 User agreement or a clear statutory mandate are the only bases of partnership-based intervention.
3 Intervention must be based on the views of all relevant family members and carers.
4 Services must be based on negotiated agreement rather than on assumptions and/or prejudices concerning the behaviour and wishes of users.
5 Users must have the greatest possible degree of choice in the services they are offered.

As the authors point out, these principles concern the authority for interventions and are aimed at working in partnership. While partnership and empowerment are not the same, partnership does, and must, involve a sharing of power. Furthermore, recent legislation clearly provides the opportunity for using partnership principles to empower users.

Foster care legislation has provided very specific guidelines for a partnership approach. Research by Sellick (1992) indicates the importance of providing adequate support to short-term carers. But the overriding theme of his study is that this support needs to be offered in partnership with carers and he concludes by providing a support checklist which, he suggests, is a tool for partnership. The checklist identifies each source of support: social work support, mutual support, support groups, training, local associations, respite, specialist support and financial support. It then lists those who should be involved in its supply and sets out the primary areas to be looked at by everyone involved in providing a foster care service to a particular child or young person.

Partnership is also vital if services are to be appropriate for black service users. They currently experience the controlling rather than the supportive aspects of legislation. If one considers the theoretical perspectives of multiracial practice then there are two which particularly involve partnership. The first is the structural position, which is a socialist/Marxist perspective. This perspective can be seen in client-centred community-based practice, which provides black communities and black users with more material resources through black community organizations. Secondly, there is the black professional perspective, which stresses ethnic identity and sharing power with black people. Practice under black direction therefore supports the strengths of black communities and is designed to meet need in ways considered appropriate by black people (Ely and Denney 1987).

Although partnership is a key principle of recent legislation it is also underpinned by familial ideology. In Chapter 3 we considered how values concerning such ideology affect legislation. This makes it all the more important to emphasize the notion of partnership and shared care as a way of facilitating families, children and young people and developing anti-oppressive practice. Consider parenting. Jordan (1990) points out that parenting is not the exclusive activity of two people carried out in their own territory. Often it is shared between a number of kin or a group of friends or an employee and employer (nurse, nanny), and involves others, such as health visitors, playgroup leaders, nursery staff or teachers, who are not usurpers of parental rights but have a complementary task in bringing up children.

Ideally social care services should be a part of this network. If we start from the premise of services being voluntarily received and supportive then parents would be encouraged to see services as assisting in their children's upbringing rather than compensating for their own perceived inadequacies – and this could include reception into care. Just as periods of living with friends are normal features of any family's supportive network, parents should be able to request periods of respite care, or even total care, be closely consulted about placement and be involved in the decision making.

Five-year-old Danny is severely brain damaged and requires round the clock medical care. His parents refused to take him home from hospital following a particularly severe epileptic fit which caused further brain damage. They felt unable to give him the care that he needed and requested that he be accommodated by the local authority. He was placed in a residential establishment managed by a voluntary agency. The residential home was only a couple of miles from where the family lived and they developed an excellent working relationship with Danny's key worker. However, the local authority considered that Danny's needs would more adequately be met within a family environment and proposed to find a foster placement for him. The parents were unhappy about this. They wanted to work in partnership with the local authority in providing for their son, whom they loved and cared about. However, they were denied access to meetings, did not understand the decision making processes and were not given information about reasons for decisions being made. They were told that they would be taken to court if they opposed the plans of the local authority. This case clearly demonstrates the clash of ideology between familial perspectives and community/shared care perspectives and the problems that can occur.

At present residential care is not considered as a positive option (Berridge 1985; Bamford and Wolkind 1988; Rowe et al. 1989). Some of the reasons for this are theoretically based, particularly with reference to familial ideologies. Thus there is an expectation that families should care for their children, and it is only if the family is perceived to have failed that the state intervenes in the form of care. This then compounds the negative views of care rather than considering it as part of a process of 'shared care'. Frost and Stein (1989) have argued that it is only by developing more flexible state support and preventive programmes that the drift towards policies which, in a divided and unequal society, act as a market transferring children to dominant class and racial groups, can be stopped. Residential care can play an important part in child care services, with residential staff being involved as key partners in the care plans.

Partnership is inspired by the belief that the most neglected resources in the current systems are the ideas and experiences of service users, members of the community, basic grade workers, home helps, etc. (Rojek *et al.* 1988). The current system allows them to express their (extremely valuable) views in an *ad hoc* way but allows no formal way of translating their ideas and experiences into policy. This not only breeds resentment and negativism but also wastes vital resources in providing relevant services: the talents and energies of people who use them.

It is also important to remember that social care agencies are 'junior partners' in terms of provision (Coulshed 1988) – relatives, friends and neighbours do most of the work. But does this raise difficulties for professionals? Is real partnership a myth? Does it really support networks without taking them over? By engaging in partnership with users and carers are professionals in effect exploiting those who feel a moral obligation to care, especially women? We would argue that partnership can and should be anti-oppressive. As Rojek *et al.* point out, partnership is not the answer to everything. Yet health and social care practitioners and carers are skilled and talented people. And these skills and talents can be used in partnership to build systems of care which are more relevant to felt needs.

Empowerment or disempowerment?

Partnership is not necessarily based on equal power relationships. Indeed the question could be asked: 'can it *ever* be based on equal power relationships?' Within the legislation there are themes of partnership and there are some guidance notes as to how to implement partnership. But as practitioners we have to be aware of the need to empower rather than disempower, and the need to balance power relationships. We will therefore go on to consider a number of ways in which a partnership approach can be managed: working with individuals, working with groups and multi-disciplinary partnerships.

Written agreements

One method of managing partnerships is through the use of written agreements (MacDonald 1991; Braye and Preston-Shoot 1992b). This method has been written into the guidance and regulations of some legislation (The Children Act 1989 Guidance and Regulations Volume 3; National Standards for the Supervision of Offenders in the Community 1992). Such agreements can be disempowering in that the partnerships are unlikely to be based on equal power relationships. Thus they may be used to control and maintain the power base of the worker. For instance, failure to comply with the supervision plan of a probation order could result in breach action under Schedule 2 to the 1991 Criminal Justice Act. In child protection work, agreements can be used as a means to ensure that parents reach a standard that has been defined by the worker as acceptable to them. If the parents fail to reach the required standards then the worker has the evidence in the form of the 'failed' agreement to take to court to prove the case against them. Setting people up to fail is by no stretch of the imagination empowering. Nor is it a recommended method of making and sustaining working relationships.

If agreements instigated by workers are to be successful then those workers have to be aware of their own value base. They also have to be able to acknowledge the power they have as workers (in terms of status and agency function) and then decide on the extent to which they are prepared to share power. Workers also have to be aware of the context of people's lives; for instance, there is no point in having an agreement which places unrealistic expectations on parents to visit their children in an establishment miles away if they are in receipt of benefits and the agency is not prepared to provide or pay for transport.

Written agreements have a better chance of working if the parties can:

- share a common understanding of the problems;
- have a degree of mutual trust;
- have a common way of expressing themselves;
- have a shared understanding of time;
- have a broadly similar view of the context in which the problems have arisen (MacDonald 1991).

The best partnerships are where the power differences are minimized and the above pointers indicate how this could be facilitated within a written agreement.

Advocacy

Advocacy as a method of working can be identified in varying forms. However, the general principles of advocacy are very much about a partnership approach. Some general points about the advocacy process will illustrate this.

- Advocates need to retain the flexibility to adapt the process to the wishes of the individual involved.
- The user should feel in control of the process and needs to trust the advocate only to take action which has been agreed.
- Advocacy is about empowerment.
- Advocacy is about supporting people to speak for themselves or presenting their views for them.
- Advocacy ensures that people are able to make informed and free choices.

- Advocacy is about advising, assisting and supporting. It is not about pres-surizing or persuading, which would then disempower.

Sometimes an advocate may need to support someone to pursue a course of action that he or she may not feel is in that person's best interests. However, since those people who need the assistance of an advocate are already in a powerless situation, often trying to have their voices heard and respected in situations where professionals have been used to keeping control and power, it is fair to say that there will be an army of professionals and interested others who will be ensuring that *their* opinions are also heard!

The advocate does not of course have to be self-sufficient and have all the answers. It is appropriate for the advocate to seek support, advice, informa-tion and assistance from others, providing that the position of the users is not compromised. The role of an advocate demands a complex mixture of skills, and challenges the traditional assumptions about the nature of the relationship between workers, carers and users. In practice it can evoke a wide range of responses, from open hostility to enthusiastic support. For that reason an advocate needs to be independent in order to function effectively.

There are many who feel that social workers, carers, health visitors, general practitioners, teachers or any person close to the user involved can be an advocate. While they may be able to use advocacy skills and on occasions advocate on behalf of someone, the context is that the process is guided by the user's agenda. The advocate only promotes the view of the user, irrespec-tive of other considerations. For example, it can be disempowering for both the user and the person acting as an advocate if they feel constrained by employers: 'those who exhibit a willingness to stand up on behalf of the people they serve, frequently find themselves in trouble with the employing body' (Kennedy 1990: 17). Carers, equally, can feel constrained by their own obligations and duties and find it difficult truly to advocate if their own needs conflict with the needs of the person they are caring for. Perhaps even more disempowering for the user is when someone appears to be acting as an advocate, and yet continues to act in her or his own role, such as social worker, nurse or probation officer. Thus it has been suggested that for pro-fessionals there are dilemmas, and to take on the advocacy role for service users who already feel powerless is likely to be as distressing for practitioners as it is for users (Barford and Wattam 1991).

One group of service users who may need an advocate are parents with learning difficulties. It would appear that many workers and carers find it difficult to work within the values of normalization when it comes to allow-ing people with learning difficulties access to the same social roles as other citizens, such as parenthood. Quite often parents with learning disabilities risk losing their children. By way of illustration we will consider the case of Mrs Peters, whose first baby was born in 1988 and then taken into care. She married shortly after and had a second child, who was made a Ward of Court. Mrs Peters had a learning difficulty. She only wanted a home of her own and for her children to be happy. Mrs Peters's parents advocated on her behalf and complained about her treatment. The local ombudsman subse-quently found that the local authority had failed to discharge its responsibility under the Children Act 1989 to provide the support and counselling she needed. Despite the emphasis on partnership with parents in the Children Act 1989, it is unlikely that the situation for parents with learning disabilities will change:

> Partnership with parents with learning difficulties must mean open-mindedness and innovation from professionals, backed up by flexible, sensitive and changing services, and changing support for parents and children so both can flourish.
>
> (Ward 1993: 23)

In summary, anti-oppressive practice with parents with learning disabilities means not only using the relevant sections of the law in relation to provision of support and counselling but also being aware of what decisions have been made in relation to different situations. Thus knowledge of the ruling in the case of Mrs Peters and of research (Booth and Booth 1994) can assist practitioners in promoting the need for particular services and so work towards changing the situation for parents with learning difficulties.

Charters

Another way of managing partnership is through the use of charters. Charters drawn up by users clearly identify their needs, which have to be taken account of by practitioners. The process of drawing up and publicizing a charter is empowering for users. But does this necessarily mean that all charters are empowering? Those drawn up by users invariably have common themes, formats and language, including rights, communication, support, consultation and partnership. They reflect their concerns, needs and demands (Bornat *et al.* 1993). An example of such a charter is the Ten-point Plan for Carers drawn up by carers' organizations supporting the King's Fund Carers' Project. Carers need:

1 *Recognition of their contribution* and of their own needs as individuals in their own right.
2 *Services tailored to their individual circumstances*, needs and views, through discussions at the time help is being planned.
3 *Services which reflect an awareness of differing racial, cultural and religious backgrounds and values*, equally accessible to carers of every race and ethnic origin.
4 *Opportunities for a break*, both for short spells (an afternoon) and for longer periods (a week or more), to relax and have time to themselves.
5 *Practical help* to lighten the tasks of caring, including domestic help, home adaptations, incontinence services and help with transport.
6 *Someone to talk to* about their own emotional needs, at the outset of caring, while they are caring and when the caring task is over.
7 *Information* about available benefits and services as well as how to cope with the particular condition of the person cared for.
8 *An income which covers the cost of caring* and which does not preclude carers taking employment or sharing care with other people.

9 *Opportunities to explore alternatives to family care*, for both the immediate and the long-term future.
10 *Services designed through consultation* with carers, at all levels of policy planning.

Charters of course are now an essential element of many public services. Six months after he became Prime Minister, John Major launched the Citizen's Charter. However, we must be careful not to assume that all charters necessarily indicate true partnership within an empowering relationship. Cooper (1993), in her analysis of the Citizen's Charter, suggests that far from being an instrument to empower citizens, various charters either are merely statements of the role of government departments or are seen as ways of facilitating the effective processing of departmental work. Thus they can be seen as a political attempt to 'depoliticize' social policy.

There are, for example, considerable differences between charters: the Council Tenant's Charter shows a greater concern for democracy than the Custom and Excise Traveller's Charter. Thus while the first imposes responsibilities on local authority housing departments to provide an efficient service to meet the needs of tenants, the reciprocal nature of the Traveller's Charter means that travellers are required to be honest in declaring goods on which customs and excise is payable. The Council Tenant's Charter has also been used as a strategic way of publicizing government policy changes, such as the right to buy and the right to choose who will carry out housing repairs, referring to the privatization of services.

The Parent's Charter is another charter fraught with difficulties. First, it assumes that all parents desire the same standards and objectives in education – those compatible with Conservative ideology. Parents have the right to complain, therefore, if the National Curriculum is not being taught, but not if they are opposed to the changes. Equally there is no commitment to teach all children about other cultures, or to provide an anti-discriminatory curriculum. Furthermore, the Charter completely denies children and young people any rights as service users or as citizens. All these observations indicate that the charters are designed to be compatible with the current political ideology. Perhaps one of the most interesting aspects of the political charters is those who are excluded from them.

Apart from young people, already mentioned in relation to the Parent's Charter, Cooper points out that currently there is no charter for residents in psychiatric institutions or for those who are homeless or mentally ill. Such charters, then, far from being empowering, can be seen to be no more than 'an autocratic instrument attempting to impose standards, and to regulate social relations within civil society's domain' (Cooper 1993: 157). Charters are not legislative instruments and although many of the standards promised may be written into statute they only reflect the dominant ideologies. Thus it is unlikely that the Citizen's Charter 'will prove empowering for those communities in Britain who need more than a change in the language of state bureaucracies or the chance to become a public sector customer to achieve meaningful citizenship' (Cooper 1993: 167). It is important to respect those charters which are user-led and can provide the basis of a partnership

approach. These, however, must not be confused with public service charters, which can be disempowering and not necessarily in the best interests
of users.

Inter-agency partnership

Partnership between agencies has been identified as an essential element of
good practice, both in the legislation and in guidelines. For some, legislation
provides the trigger for closer working relations. A project in Wigan to divert
young people away from court was assisted by the introduction of the Criminal Justice Act 1991. Social workers and probation officers, who had previously been working together, were enabled by the legislation to pressurize
for an inter-agency team. The 'juvenile justice team' subsequently set up
consisted of social workers and probation officers working together to provide
a more flexible seamless service. Obviously such a partnership requires discussions on aims, values and the need to produce joint policy statements.
But it also widens the pool of resources and skills available to provide the
service needed.

The arrival of 'care packages' and 'multi-disciplinary care management',
particularly as a result of the community care legislation, has meant that
agencies have had to develop partnership strategies. However, attitudes between health and social services are epitomized by the inter-professional
rivalry which stems from different approaches to service provision. Differences in professional ethics, accountability, standards and resources also characterize the relationship. It is for this reason, perhaps, that the document
Working Together (DoH 1991a) was produced by government departments.
The aim was to facilitate inter-professional and inter-agency cooperation
and so to enable local authorities to work in partnership with parents and
children in protecting children from abuse. It stresses the need for social
services departments, police, medical practitioners, community health workers,
schools, voluntary organizations and any other concerned parties to develop
close working relationships. This can be achieved through recognized joint
forums in the form of area child protection committees. What the document
states as essential is that committee procedures provide a mechanism to
enable agencies to share information with other agencies wherever one agency
becomes concerned that a child may be at risk. This guidance is actually
issued under Section 7 of the Local Authority Social Services Act 1970, which,
while not having the full force of statute, should be complied with 'unless
local circumstances indicate exceptional reasons which justify a variation'
(DoH 1991a: iii).

Planning services

It makes sense that those who need and use services should have a say in
those services – not only in what services they require, but also in how they
are delivered and who delivers them. But traditionally, in both statutory and
voluntary agencies, the service providers have seen themselves somehow as
official protectors of vulnerable people and so, despite legislation recognizing

the need for empowerment and participation and the genuine commitment of many service providers to involve people who use their services, problems abound.

In 1991 a series of workshops involving users and providers looked at how to break down some of the barriers that exist and why user involvement can be problematic. The account of these workshops, *Building Bridges* (Harding 1993), recognized that there is a history of distrust and unequal power relationships between users of services and those who provide them. In order for any initiative to be successful users need to be able to build self-confidence, solidarity and strength through working together in groups. Even so, they still do not have the same resources, paid time, access to training or credibility of 'professionals' and their views are often devalued. Clearly this imbalance has to be addressed if an equal partnership is to be achieved.

In describing her work in the Action Research Project in Honiton and other parts of Devon, Bryan (1990) notes that physically disabled young people or those who care for them rarely feel empowered by existing service provision. She argues that empowering users means allowing them true participation by regarding them as colleagues in the participative process. How can we do this? It has been suggested that before reaching out to involve users of services, workers should ask four questions (Wallcraft 1990).

The first is: *why involve users?* For those who feel that they *ought to* because it is in the legislation or the current trend, then the hurdle here is to consider the problems and benefits of sharing power with people who have been systematically disempowered in the past.

The next question is: *who do you want to involve?* If it is only those *hand picked* because they will make a positive contribution then there is no real commitment to power sharing and the most that will happen is the creation of a new elite group.

The third question is: *who are you not reaching?* Women may not use the service unless there is a women-only space and provision for their children. Black people may find the service inappropriate and unwelcoming. Access may not be possible for people with disabilities.

The final question to be asked is: *what are you offering?* True user involvement is not about asking how the place should be decorated. The extent of user involvement must be honestly assessed – is it consultation or a direct say in decisions? Unrealistic expectations are raised if there is a lack of honesty about how far providers are prepared to go in power sharing.

Many organizations exclude people through their structures of formal meetings, use of language and pre-set objectives (Harding 1993), so that they are left feeling like *ignorant outsiders* with no notion of how to get their ideas considered or even how to get elected on to the committee (Wallcraft 1990). There is no doubt that surrendering power, particularly if this involves surrendering control over financial and other resources, and involves working against the grain of your employing organization, is considered to be a risky business (Wallcraft 1990; Harding 1993). It can also be stressful for workers as 'they juggle conflicting values' (Harding 1993). These are similar to dilemmas identified for people drawing up working agreements.

For some, getting a user perspective on those who hold the power to affect change involves developing campaigning organizations. *Awaaz* (meaning 'inner voice') is a project in Manchester which has developed in response to the lack of services for members of the Asian community who have had negative experiences of psychiatric services. It acts as a resource by providing information and advice on a range of mental health issues. It works on the premise that if it can raise awareness about black mental health issues and change attitudes then this will eventually affect the delivery of services. Services within the project are based on needs and experiences as relayed by the users. One of the achievements of the project has been to support a black users' group in the local day hospital, where hospital staff are invited every three weeks to hear and respond to suggestions and grievances. *Awaaz* is also developing advocacy projects. Through these projects the gaps and inequalities in the provision of services for Asian people are highlighted.

A notional partnership exists in the funding, in that the group was funded by a one year starter grant from social services, but clearly long-term funding and resources are needed for groups such as this to function effectively. However, both central and local government have powers to work in partnership with local groups to respond in this way to the needs and experiences of users in the planning and provision of services. Anti-oppressive practice means knowing what powers there are to provide resources in this way and also knowing how to apply for such funding.

A similar argument has been used to encourage the development of organizations controlled by disabled people. Morris (1993a) cites a number of examples of projects which have successfully demonstrated ways in which services controlled by disabled people create opportunities for independent living. However, the government, health authorities and social services departments must work in partnership with organizations of disabled people in purchasing services under the contracting arrangements. Such organizations are essential to the development of services which disabled people want. Morris suggests that putting resources into such organizations and enabling the voice of service users to be heard at all stages of community care implementation should help to bring about the shift needed from service-led to resource-led provision.

Involving users in partnership and the planning of services should also mean involving them in the selection and appointment of staff. This is a logical extension of the obligation of local authorities to consult on community care. Many voluntary agencies now involve users in recruitment but it is unusual in the statutory sector. Obviously it is important for users to receive training and to be prepared for what can be a difficult and intimidating task, even for those experienced in the process. But it also needs training input for professionals in user participation. Groups such as People First have been involved in interviews for workers in various London boroughs. People First is an organization run by users with learning difficulties. However, they refuse to be involved unless their members are taken seriously. Following a number of occasions where their views were not taken into account they now actively challenge tokenistic invitations to be on panels.

Final thoughts

True partnership means taking account of the power differentials and understanding the need to relinquish power. Partnership is an evolving, negotiated process. It does not just *happen*, you have to work at it.

Activities

Activity 1

Partnerships, as we have said, need to be worked at. Think of a situation where: (a) a partnership would be difficult; (b) a partnership would be impossible; and (c) a partnership is ideal. This could be either in your work situation or within your personal experience. Write down your feelings about each of these situations. In particular think about the following areas:

• What would make you feel good and positive about the partnership?
• What makes you feel uncomfortable and why?
• What would make you feel undermined or threatened by the partnership?

Think about your answers to this exercise and refer back to them as you work through the following scenario.

Activity 2

Jennifer is 14 years old. She has a younger brother, David, who is nine years old, and a sister, Anna, who is four years old. Jennifer's mother, Sheila, is a single parent. Jennifer's father died three years ago. During the past six months, according to Sheila, relations between herself and her daughter have deteriorated and they have been arguing on a daily basis. Jennifer has, during this period, been seen by a number of people in the community with a young man who is said to be in his twenties.

Recently, Jennifer has been staying out late – this fact has infuriated Sheila, who is concerned about her daughter's moral welfare. Sheila has accused her daughter of being lazy and selfish. Jennifer in turn believes that her mother excludes her and has more time for her younger siblings. Jennifer has at times, after a row with her mother, gone to stay with her maternal grandmother, who lives some distance away from the family home. While there, Jennifer does not attend school on a regular basis.

You are a worker involved with the family to try to improve the situation for Jennifer and ensure her regular attendance at school. Draw up a partnership agreement on the basis of the information with which you have been provided.

Commentary
Did you, in devising the agreement: consider issues of race, culture, religion and language; consult everyone in the scenario? If there was someone you left out, or did not feel was appropriate, please give your reasons for this.

If Jennifer wishes to stay with her grandmother what part of the Children Act would you use? Would any action you took affect any partnership arrangements?

- How do you attempt to sustain and promote contact between Jennifer, her family, friends and the community?
- How do you promote Jennifer's welfare?
- How would a working agreement empower the people in this situation?
- There is a potential for working agreements to disempower service users. What are the elements in this case that could be misused?

Activity 3

Jennifer's school is committed to working in partnership with parents. They write to Sheila expressing their concern about the fact that Jennifer's exams are approaching and her attendance has been problematic. They feel that she could do well but as she has missed a substantial amount of time at school she is unlikely to achieve her full potential. The following is an account of the meeting from Jennifer's perspective:

> I had to go to this meeting and I was really scared. I hadn't been to school for a while and I thought maybe they wanted to chuck me out. I wasn't sure who was going to be there apart from Mum, my year teacher and the head. My friend Janie said that when she went to a meeting her social worker was there and some other people that she'd never ever seen before.
>
> I really wanted to go to the meeting because I knew it was important, but when it came to it I had a row with my Mum and went off on my own for a walk. But then after I calmed down I decided to go in anyway. I knocked on the door and went in to the room. I looked round – I saw my Mum and someone asked me to take a seat. People just carried on talking and never even said hello. I wanted to say something but wasn't asked. Mum said a few things about the problems at home and about my boyfriend. I felt really upset and angry. I just had to say something – and did. I was told that everyone needed to have their say and they were trying to sort something out for me. But I just wanted them to listen to what I had to say.
>
> I didn't feel they really involved me in the meeting at all. At the end the social worker came up to me and said she was glad I had turned up as it was important for me to be involved.

- What do you think are the key issues if service users are to be involved in meetings?
- Do you think that the professionals involved were committed to a partnership approach?
- What could have been done differently?

6 MINIMAL

INTERVENTION

It's nice to know somebody cares
Who is interested in my welfare
A person who is always there.
Sometimes I want my freedom:
Do things for myself,
A chance to learn.
Why don't they encourage me
Instead of doing everything for me?
They don't think I am capable.
Maybe they are too scared.
Give me some responsibility
and let me make decisions.
I know I'm in a wheelchair –
but I can do things from there.

(Chrissie Elms Bennett 1994)

Thelma Lewis had suffered mental disturbance for 15 years before she was found wandering the streets naked. The body of her handicapped daughter Beverley lay emaciated in a strange house which had become their fortress, stuffed with debris like a concrete representation of the chaos of Ms Lewis' mind.

(Jervis 1989: 22)

Beverley Lewis was born blind, deaf, with learning difficulties as a result of rubella. Although it was considered that Thelma Lewis did not welcome intervention, it was apparent that the bond between mother and daughter and Thelma's devotion to her daughter were never in question. Beverley died, starved, naked and in conditions of squalor following inadequate care by her mother, who was subsequently diagnosed as suffering from schizophrenia and admitted to a psychiatric hospital. One of Ms Lewis's daughters had been told that her mother's disturbed behaviour 'was normal for someone from Jamaica' (Jervis 1989: 22). Thelma was an informal carer who herself needed care as her own condition deteriorated. 'Beverley was strangled in a web of ideology which has been woven to get the "nanny state" out of our lives' (Morgan 1989).

The case of Beverley Lewis graphically brings to our attention the issues we face in discussions about intervention into people's lives: care in the community, compulsory treatment, the strain upon carers, the problems faced by health and welfare agencies in providing appropriate coordinated services, and the application of relevant legislation in directing effective intervention strategies. Commentators at the time of the death of Beverley Lewis focused on the issue of civil liberties and the fact that while those of Thelma Lewis were preserved her daughter's were sacrificed – to the extent of her losing her life.

It is therefore impossible to talk about minimal intervention in any meaningful way without first discussing:

• the role of the state;
• our relationship as workers to the state;
• our relationship to those we are involved with – are they clients, patients, service users, consumers, welfare citizens, deserving poor, undeserving poor or just people we work with?

We will briefly explore each of these three areas in turn, which should lead us to an understanding of how and when, as either professionals or carers, we intervene in the lives of others.

The role of the state

Citizenship, according to Claire Ungerson, is always concerned with the relationship between individuals and the state: 'it is concerned with how the individual and the state relate to each other across public concerns and how public institutions, such as the judiciary and the polity, mediate that relationship' (Ungerson 1993: 143). It is perhaps helpful, therefore, to trace the concept of citizenship in an attempt to gain some understanding of the role of the state in health and social care practice.

The idea of citizenship has a long and distinguished history. It is a contested and disputed concept – different groups, all with different interests, have claimed the term. Today, citizenship still has connotations of empowerment, membership and rights, yet historically citizenship has carried with it another powerful set of values and ideas: exclusion, obligation and duty. We only have to look at the treatment of Gypsies (known as browns) within the Czech Republic and, nearer home, travellers, to see how the socially constructed term of citizenship can be used to maintain the privileges of one group over another. *What about Beverley and Thelma Lewis?* Were they considered to be full citizens with equal rights? Or were they excluded on the grounds of 'race', disability or mental health?

Within health and social care practice clients, patients or users are viewed as citizens who have paid for services either directly or indirectly, and to whom the provider of services should be accountable. This emphasis on rights is part of a consumerist trend within many public services, such as health, education and housing. Supported by central and local government policies, public services have attempted to be more accountable to those who use the services – citizens' charters have been put forward as an embodiment of this striving to be accountable.

The late 1980s and early 1990s saw a reactivation of interest in the idea of citizenship. It had emerged as a key concept at the time of the creation of the welfare state. William Beveridge acknowledged the central significance of citizenship in his report 50 years ago and it emerges once again as we seem to be moving into a post welfare state age. In our discussions about partnership we looked at the use of charters as a means of managing a partnership approach. Charters (according to Croft and Beresford 1992) can be directly linked to two factors: the growth of social movements, e.g. within lesbian and gay communities or in disability forums; and the political colon-izing by the New Right of basic socialist ideals. The charters publicize and make visible the demands of marginalized disempowered groups. The per-sonal becomes political and public – the instrument by which demands of certain welfare and social rights and expectations are met.

However, some commentators argue differently. An example of this is the Black Community Care Charter, which was produced by the National Asso-ciation of Race Equality Advisors to remind institutions of the need to in-clude a black perspective. The Children Act 1989 states that the race and culture of children and young people must be addressed in the provision of services, the guidance notes to the NHS and Community Care Act 1990 states that in the production of community care plans the needs of black people must be taken into account. The Black Community Care Charter aims to ensure that these obligations are met by the government. Coote (1992: 15), though, states that 'when the rhetoric is sorted from the substance, the Citizen's Charter offers little in the way of entitlements that can be enforced by individual citizens'. This is because 'charters are chiefly concerned to promote a market in welfare services with more private sector providers and more individual choice – yet with no regard for individuals' unequal power to choose'.

Not all charters have just emerged as a result of grass roots action by dis-possessed groups. They have emerged from centralized bureaucratic bodies – 'the product of ministerial heads produced by those who have power for those who do not' (Cooper 1993: 93). Major's charter is based on a public sector market of goods and services. It assumes that the citizen is free to have access to the services available. This is where the true contradiction between empowerment and current reality rests. Citizenship is grounded in the use of public services. But after 15 years of Conservative policies very little re-mains in the market place. No responsibility for inadequate service provision is taken by the government – it is left to the consumer to shop wisely and seek out the bargains.

The welfare citizen is defined by community care legislation as someone who is in need of services. However, community care systems, services and resources are fixed and finite. Service users' needs, we are told, should be taken into account when practitioners draw up care plans, but account has to be taken of what is available and affordable. The task, then, or, more appropriately, the challenge set for health and social care practitioners is to manage to fit the welfare citizen into market-led services.

A response to market-led services is the development of the *contract culture*. However, a Rowntree-sponsored report, *Contracting for Care*, reported that all but two of the social service departments surveyed said that contracts had done 'nothing to increase users' choice of services' (Common and Flynn 1992). In short, cutbacks and Conservative ideological policies do not provide the background for the development of public services that are aimed at breaking down the barriers of social inequalities and enhancing choice.

Citizenship, then, is not a politically neutral term. Its heritage is disputed. The left and right have made concentrated attempts to own and control the term. It is important, therefore, as health and social care practitioners and carers, that we have an understanding of what the term means to us, for it defines our relationship with both colleagues and service users.

Our relationship as workers to the state

How we interpret government legislation in the form of the policies and procedures which guide our practice will be very much dependent on how we view our relationship as workers to the state. If we consider the situation for health and social care practitioners we will find that there have been numerous debates about the role fulfilled by them within contemporary society. Are they merely an extension of the state-social police: there to maintain stability and moral order? Or is the role of the caring professions that of enabling individuals to reach their full potential? Is it the role of practitioners to make public the private experience of inequality and so be part of the process of change? Should medical practitioners, social workers, community nurses, psychiatrists and education staff have intervened in the lives of Beverley and Thelma Lewis?

The past years of economic recession, and 15 years of a Conservative government, the introduction of legislation such as the Children Act 1989, the National Health Service and Community Care Act 1990 and the Criminal Justice Act 1991, have informed the work that is carried out by health and welfare agencies. They have also placed increasing demands on workers. Spending cuts and privatization policies have added to the complexity of the relationship between health and social care practitioners and the state. Debates following the death of Beverley Lewis focused on the need for social work, medical and nursing professions to work together. The problems, responsibilities and needs that result from hospital closures have not been addressed, another issue highlighted by the death of Beverley Lewis. Public inquiries and investigations into social tragedies have in turn blamed health and welfare practitioners either for failing to intervene or for being over-zealous in their interventions into the private sphere of family life. Social workers have been subject to political and media pressure to respond to the behaviour of young offenders, who in the eyes of society are being treated too leniently for their misdemeanours. There appears to be a 'drive to press social workers into assuming a more coercive and interventionist role in policing deviant families' (Langan and Lee 1989: 3), and in particular *irresponsible* single parents. The increasing orientation of social and health welfare agencies to the needs of a market economy has meant that success is based on measurable outcomes, which places additional burdens on the worker.

The growth of active, campaigning user groups representing those who have not traditionally benefited from the health and welfare services has also affected the work of social care agencies. Such groups have developed as a result of the impact of policies, procedures and practices which have not taken account of the needs of all individuals who make up the diverse society that we live in. All the factors outlined have led to professionals having to rethink their relationship to the state and, in turn, how they should intervene in people's lives.

Our relationship to others

It is important, as we have stated in previous chapters, that we are continually aware of the impact that the personal values we hold have on our practice. Personal reflection and an understanding of the theoretical frameworks that have been offered to explain what is meant by social care are the precursors to any action that we take.

The quality and type of intervention should be based on our understanding of the relationship that exists between practitioners and users. If we view relationships in terms of an *us* and *them* perspective – where all the power resides in *us* by virtue of our professional status and our access to resources – then our interventions will not be based on empowerment. If our interventions are informed by a belief in partnership and empowerment, then we maximize the effectiveness of intervention with minimum intrusion into people's lives.

The language that we use to describe the people with whom we are working characterizes the nature of the relationship and in turn how we will intervene in their lives. Language is not neutral (Croft and Beresford 1993). It reflects the power differentials that exist within society. Dale Spender (1980), for example, has argued from a feminist perspective that in fact language is *man made*. Language conveys personal, structural and ideological messages (Phillipson 1992). The term *client* has been criticized because of its implied inequality and separateness, and other terms such as *service user* and *consumer* have entered our language. *Clients* may also be *patients* to practitioners based in the health professions; to others they will be *consumers* of purchased services (Payne 1994a).

However, such terms can also convey certain ideologies and reinforce separateness. For instance, use of the terms *carers*, *caring* and *dependent people* can have a massive impact on how such people are perceived. People who need help with their daily living activities cannot receive the respect and autonomy they should have if they are regarded as *dependent* people. Equally, their personal relationships cannot be respected if their partner, parent or relative is treated as a *carer*. Therefore it has been suggested that we need to reclaim the word *caring* to mean caring *about* someone rather than caring *for*, with 'its custodial overtones' (Morris 1993a: 174). Use of the term *citizen* has been preferred by some writers, as it has been seen to emphasize civil rights rather than refer to people in relation to service provision (Croft and Beresford 1993). However, the term citizen has also been linked with racist immigration policies and thus will always have a negative impact on black communities who already experience discrimination.

In our intervention, therefore, we have to be aware of the way in which language can reflect power differentials and have an impact on people with whom we are working. This means using the words that people themselves understand and the words by which they wish to define themselves. The language of health and welfare has been said to be a form of power (Rojek *et al.* 1988). It enables workers to label others and define what is acceptable and unacceptable behaviour. Terms such as *disturbed*, *at risk* and *in need* describe behaviour from a particular value perspective.

Links to practice: Beverley Lewis

Let us look back at the case of Beverley Lewis and consider some of these issues. The state provided the legislative framework within which intervention could have been facilitated. Despite criticisms of the lack of available legislative powers at the time, this appeared to focus on the need for compulsory powers rather than a consideration of the preventive measures available. The lack of appropriate intervention could be attributed to racism within society, attitudes about the privacy of the family, and the protection and control of vulnerable people. What were the dilemmas posed to professionals by this case? We can begin to answer this by posing the following questions:

- Were the practitioners supposed to act as guardians to Beverley?
- Were the practitioners supposed to respect Thelma's wishes in refusing intervention?
- Does Beverley have the right to intervention against the wishes of her mother?
- Were the practitioners supposed to maintain this family and support Thelma as a carer – bearing in mind the close bond between them (as the coroner commented, to have separated Beverley from her mother would not have been in her best interests)?
- Should the focus have been merely on these two people or on assistance given to the wider family and community networks to support the mother in the face of her hostility to statutory intervention?
- Should people deemed to be schizophrenic have the right to look after their own children?

• Should support services be based on the carer's needs rather than the person cared for or vice versa?

The story of Beverley Lewis sadly indicates the problems of intervening appropriately in the lives of vulnerable people. Workers were given the power to intervene, which could have enabled Beverley Lewis to live a fuller life. The practitioners in this case appeared to see the law as a stumbling block rather than a vehicle for change. Because they considered that they had no *powers* to intervene they were able to claim that they had no *duty* to intervene. But ethically they had obligations. At the end of the day *no action at all* can be as oppressive as intrusion into people's lives. It has been said that if there are high quality and reliable support services then private care, in the context of a strong bond between two people, can be supported within state provision of care (Ungerson 1993).

When to intervene?

Intervention can be identified on three levels: primary, secondary and tertiary (Herbert 1993). This has been identified in relation to working within child protection but can be transferred to all user groups who require services.

The *primary level* is effectively preventive, i.e. acknowledging that problems exist and putting in services to minimize risk and harm. Within this there are three main approaches, which we will illustrate with reference to a project for young people whose parents are identified as problem drinkers.

1 *Adapting existing services.* Often young people whose parents are problem drinkers are young carers. This means that once they are home from school their time is taken up looking after themselves, and often their parents, as well as managing the household tasks. The project therefore provides a facility, in conjunction with the education department, where young people can do their homework within school hours. This strategy has a significant impact on the education of young people whose home lives are disrupted by their parents' drinking patterns. It also gives them the confidence to discuss their difficulties without the very real fear many young carers have of intrusive intervention, which could result in their reception into care.
2 *Mobilization of community resources.* The project provides telephone help lines and access to counsellors for young people. A drop-in centre also operates where the focal point is the cafe area which provides cheap nutritious meals. This not only provides the young people with the opportunity to eat a hot meal but also is a meeting place where they can talk and share experiences.
3 *Education of the public.* The project does this by publicizing the service for young people and through publicity campaigns brings the problem of young people in such a situation into the public and professional arena. While the publicity targeted at the young people who are troubled by their circumstances is specific it can also motivate the parents to seek help.

Secondary intervention is about the reduction of existing problems through early detection and intervention. Herbert (1993) uses the example of offering services to identified *high-risk* families who are in need of help in coping with their children to avoid serious harm. As Parton (1985: 192) points out, 'the emphasis should be on assisting parents to manage their children rather than monitoring or constraining them'.

Tertiary intervention occurs after the investigation of serious incidents, e.g. after a compulsory admission under the mental health legislation or any form of abuse of either children or adults. The aim is to reduce the adverse effects of the incident by provision of appropriate services.

The concept of minimal intervention is enshrined in legislation; for example, in the Children Act (Section 1(5)).

> Where a court is considering whether or not to make one or more orders under this Act with respect to a child, it shall not make the order or any of the orders unless it considers that doing so would be better for the child than making no order at all.

However, as Braye and Preston-Shoot (1992a) point out, the law does not provide the answers as to when or how to intervene and thus a practice as well as a legal rationale is needed for intervention. Furthermore, intervention occurs at individual, family, group, organizational, community and societal levels and requires the ability to use effectively a range of skills and methods at varying times (DuBois and Krogsgrud Miley 1992).

Perhaps the most severe form of intervention is the compulsory removal from home of both children and adults. Stevenson (1989) points out that the justification of compulsory removal from home is that the person concerned is at risk because:

- of their own actions;
- of the actions of others;
- they are placing others at risk.

She suggests that these risks fall into five basic categories.

1 Physical injury or neglect. The focus has primarily been on children in the past but elder abuse is now being increasingly recognized as an area of concern.
2 Those considered to be at risk either socially or emotionally (rather than physically). It is difficult to define such abuse and the danger of white middle-class values being imposed on the recipients of social care services in such situations is very real. It is, however, possible to intervene in the lives of children and young people in such situations using child care law, but there are no legislative powers for adults.
3 Those who are a physical risk to others in the immediate environment which the behaviour of the individual may occasion. While it is more usual in the case of mentally ill adults, this can include children and young people alleged to be uncontrollable by their carers, or older people who may perhaps be aggressive towards a partner.
4 Social risk. Young offenders can easily be identified in this category and can be seen as a risk to the community in terms of the breakdown of law

and order rather than any physical risk (unless the offences are violent or endanger life). Stevenson suggests that this category is more open to exploitation by those with power, particularly in the case of young people.

5 Environmental risk. This is where the lifestyle of an individual causes problems for others; for example, where squalid living conditions lead to infestation, causing health hazards to others in the community.

Braye and Preston-Shoot (1992a: 56) point to the need for a framework for decision making, which they say is both a 'safety device and a moral imperative'. Such a framework, they say, provides for consistency of practice and consists of three parts.

1 *Structure*. This is a series of questions which can be used to assist judgement. They may be asked of service users, colleagues, managers or themselves and come under the headings of what, when, who and how?

2 *Substance*. This is essentially a combination of theory, knowledge and practice wisdom which informs the decision making process. In particular, Braye and Preston-Shoot cite examples of checklists which can be used to appraise a situation. Government guidance in some instances promotes the use of checklists to assist in the implementation of legislation, such as in child protection assessments (DoH 1988) and the Mental Health Code of Practice (DoH 1990).

3 *Principles*. These are the values which underpin the decision making processes.

A framework for decision making has to take into account a number of factors. In particular it has to provide for legal knowledge and social work practice wisdom to work together. Of course it is not easy to do this and to use the law positively. As Braye and Preston-Shoot point out, the lack of precision over definitions and the power it thus gives to professionals means that there are many different interpretations that can be made. In using the law positively, however, to promote anti-oppressive practice and to minimize intervention in people's lives, it is important to make informed decisions.

Brayne and Martin (1990: 166), in discussing investigation in child protection, consider the vital words in the legislation to be 'safeguarding and promoting the welfare of the child'. Safeguarding and promoting, they say, are 'positive words', whereas inaction is 'rarely positive' (p. 170). The dilemmas for those investigating arise because of the tensions between outcomes. As Stevenson (1989: 162) points out, 'although the decision concerning the extent of injury or neglect which justifies removal might be contentious, the underlying principle that, in certain circumstances, children must be protected from physical harm caused by their caretakers is not'. But those involved in an investigation will be involved in trying to balance societal demands and the needs of the young person. In the light of this Brayne and Martin (1990: 167) suggest that practitioners will always be involved in the following issues.

• Therapeutic intervention, i.e. trying to help the young person (which can be achieved through using various powers, duties and services).
• Statutory control. Using the courts and statutory powers to produce evidence that the grounds for an order are satisfied.

• Prosecuting the perpetrator. In the case of murder of a child prosecution
is acceptable. In the case of abuse the situation is more difficult and thus
'investigating the facts with the child and the child's family for this particular end, whilst still trying to give therapeutic support becomes even
harder'.

It is important to remember that the 'aim of the investigation must be to
establish what help, support and services may be offered, and also to consider whether there will be a need for court proceedings' (Brayne and Martin
1990: 168).

When the information has been gathered a decision has to be made as to
how to intervene. Braye and Preston-Shoot's model for decision making
offers the chance for legal knowledge and practice wisdom to operate together. Such a framework is necessary to 'fully provide for the subtleties of
the situations social workers face in applying the law, [and] for the multi-
plicity of influences upon the process' (Braye and Preston-Shoot 1992a: 63).

Use of various legislation can of course maximize or minimize intervention. In January 1993 Ben Silcock, a schizophrenic, was mauled after attempting to share his New Year's Eve lunch with the lions at London Zoo.
Ben lived alone by choice in a council flat. His family were supportive and
regularly helped him. The day hospital only provided short-term support
and the local centre run by the charity MIND banned him after he had hit
a member of staff. There are a number of dilemmas in this case in terms of
decision making and the degree of intervention:

• whether medication should be used to control the condition;
• if a person is living in the community, whether she or he should be forced
  to take medication;
• when people should be admitted for compulsory treatment in hospital.

The response of the Health Secretary, Virginia Bottomley, was to call for a
review of the 1983 Mental Health Act, proposing more compulsory powers
to detain and treat discharged patients.

The Royal College of Psychiatrists proposed a system of Community Supervision Orders which have caused widespread debate. Such proposals, it has
been argued, would offer only limited choices to patients, i.e. they can either
agree to treatment in the community or return to hospital. However, Mrs
Silcock, when writing about her experiences in 1993, pointed out that the
care team would have right of access to the person concerned and so be
more able to use persuasion. There is general agreement that some of the
College's proposals were vague. However, the issues are about compulsory
treatment. Mrs Silcock asked whether preventive compulsory treatment would
be 'so terrible' if, without treatment in the community, people deteriorate
and end up in hospital, with their freedom curtailed, their choices limited
and their frustrations increased.

Organizations such as MIND argue that the adverse effects of medication
can be distressing and that the kind of supervision suggested by the College
could be provided through guardianship, which to date has been very
little used under the Mental Health Act 1983. However Mrs Silcock points

out that guardianship is often regarded as toothless because it has no power to enforce medication. While compulsory powers are not an attractive proposition, she argues that if all else fails they should be seen as an option, but one which is part of a dedicated care programme, which must have built-in safeguards to prevent abuse.

The fear of infringing civil liberties is at the heart of the controversy about levels of intervention concerning the care of people like Ben Silcock. As Ian Bynoe, Legal Director of MIND, said at the time, 'assuming discharged patients are capable of living in the community means allowing them to take risks, subject to intervention under the Mental Health Act'. With Ben, when he stopped taking medication his mental state deteriorated. His mother has said that 'not taking the drugs made him feel powerful; it made him feel part of a colourful world which was far more exciting than real life'. One could argue that we all have a right to choose a life that we find exciting – and if the real world for us was deadened by drugs, then perhaps we too would choose not to take them. The problems occur when we threaten either our own life or the lives of other people. And so we inevitably come back to the question of when, and how, to intervene. And, perhaps more importantly, do we intervene in an oppressive way or do we find the resources to intervene in a way that is not oppressive or dangerous?

With Ben Silcock, as with Thelma Lewis, there was talk of lack of legislative powers. MIND, among others, believes that the legislation already provides for intervention by professionals when necessary and thus any further powers would be oppressive. For instance, a man with a history like Ben Silcock's can be detained in hospital for treatment under Section 3 of the Mental Health Act 1989, and can, under Paragraph 2.9 of the Code of Practice to the Act, be detained if there is a known history of mental illness following the refusal to take medication. Duties under Section 117 on aftercare apply to people for whom a Community Supervision Order is suggested.

MIND feels that such duties could be clarified by statutory directions on how to assess on discharge from hospital and the obligations of social services departments under Section 47 of the NHS and Community Care Act 1990. Section 7 of the Act (guardianship) provides powers of supervision for agencies, so what is needed, says MIND, is properly organized community supervision. Debates in cases such as these are necessary so that legislation does not become more oppressive, and indicate how important it is for practitioners and carers to understand the scope of powers under the law. They can then use the law to promote anti-oppressive practice, which should include ensuring that relatives are made aware of their rights within the legislation.

Within these debates, as with Thelma and Beverley Lewis, we must remember the people concerned. So many professionals and interested parties have an opinion. But often those about whom the debates range have no one to represent them. This is clearly where the need for independent advocacy is paramount. An independent advocate does not have to consider the interests of anyone except the person with whom she or he is working.

Ben Silcock wanted to live an independent life – he lived alone by choice. One has to be careful in implementing legislation that any intervention does not cause people to become so dependent that the provision in itself then becomes oppressive, however forward thinking it might be. For instance, Morris (1993a) demonstrates in her research that care in the community can often create dependency and that it is merely a new form of institutionalization within the community. She particularly looks at imaginative ways of giving users choice and power by enabling them to control their own finances, which then gives them the power to purchase resources. Use of monies from the Independent Living Fund (ILF) was one example.

Paula had been sexually and physically abused by her father for as long as she could remember. By applying for money from the ILF and with help from a housing association she was able to leave this situation and move into a place of her own. Morris says: 'In contrast to the institutionalisation created by statutory services and the dependency created by informal care, those who employed their own helpers were able to participate in social and personal relationships, and some were also in paid employment' (Morris 1993a: 23). She quotes Jack Talbot, who simply said:

> I'm a husband, a father, and a breadwinner. Ten years ago I was in an institution where I couldn't even decide when I would go to the toilet. You know, you can't really understand it if you haven't done it. Your whole life changes.
>
> (Morris 1993a: 23)

Morris reminds us that direct payments to individuals can be made without breaking the law, by the setting up of a trust or by the use of voluntary organizations to administer grants for personal assistance. The government has indicated that social services departments should not make payments to individuals. However, there is increasing evidence that giving people cash to manage and control the care that they require is more enabling, creates a better quality of life and is more cost-effective than statutory provision. As in any empowerment strategy, the opportunities can only be maximized if they are part of the process of empowerment. This means that service users must also have access to advocacy, advice and assistance and the support of other disabled people who had similar experiences in employing their own personal assistance.

What is acceptable risk?

As carers and as practitioners we live with risk every day. The art is in deciding what is acceptable. Bradshaw et al. provide a solution based on provision of choices.

> The danger of active interventionist policies to ensure that aid is brought quickly to those who collapse is that such policies may interfere with the lives and deaths of those who prefer to remain at home. This is not intended to imply that no action should be taken, but rather that social policy should aim to provide a valid choice. The elderly should be free to choose whether or not to live alone. If they have been bereaved of relatives and friends they should be enabled to develop new social contacts if they so desire. If they are at risk of sudden collapse they should

be informed of this, and if they wish to they should be provided with the opportunity to make use of good neighbour schemes, alarm systems or telephone schemes. These services and facilities should be made available to old people so that they can make a reasoned choice. For such a choice to be meaningful, it must be based on accurate information as to what services are available, and on a wide range of alternatives, ranging from shared living schemes to telephone checks.

(Bradshaw *et al.* 1978; quoted in Tinker 1981)

Judgements are made according to our own value position, our experiences and available facts. Our decision to act is based on how we interpret a given situation, which in turn guides our level of intervention. In considering risk the issues of *rights* and *harm* have to be balanced. This balance is about recognizing what power we have rather than being patronizing and over-protective. It is also about ensuring that everyone involved has access to necessary information. For those who are unable to articulate their needs it is about ensuring that they have someone who can act as an advocate. The *assessment* of risk, therefore, is no easy task and needs to be made in *partnership* with all concerned.

Final thoughts

It could be argued that the use of the word intervention is oppressive and by its very nature indicates where the power base lies. Given such an observation perhaps a more useful way of describing the process could be that *interaction* takes place rather than intervention. This then reminds us that we should be working in partnership and are less likely to be accused of either violating rights or, at the other end of the spectrum, neglect. This is not to legitimize a vague and unfocused approach to the work that we do, but reminds us to think about such work and how we can promote anti-oppressive practice. Of course it can equally be argued that to call the process interaction is dishonest in situations of compulsion, and that the word *intervention* more accurately reflects what is happening. To describe the process as inter-action would only be relevant, therefore, in cases of *minimal* intervention. The language used conveys the type of relationship that the worker has with the service user – it relates to the practice that is carried out. This is an area of continuing debate that is something for you to consider.

Activity

1 How would you define risk?
2 Think of three situations where you have consciously taken a risk. What were the advantages of doing so? What were the disadvantages?
3 Do you feel that vulnerable people should be allowed to live in conditions that are hazardous to their health and place them in danger if they refuse help?
4 Should residential care be used to protect people from risk at the cost of depriving them of their liberty?

5 How can vulnerable people prevent medical treatment from being forced upon them?

Under Section 8 of the Children Act 1989 young people who are of a sufficient age and understanding have the right to refuse medical treatment. Look at the following law reports:

Gillick v *West Norfolk and Wisbech AHA* [1986] AC 112.
Re J (a Minor) (Inherent Jurisdiction: Consent to Treatment) [1992] *The Times* 15 July.
Re R (a Minor) (Wardship: Consent to Treatment) [1992] Fam 11.
R v *Kirklees MBC ex parte C (a Minor)* [1992] 2 FLR 117.

The issues in all these cases concern the rights of young people to determine what medical treatment they should accept. When reading through the reports think about the following points.

• Do you feel that the courts were justified in the decisions made?
• How have the issues of rights and harm been balanced?
• Were the decisions made from a protectionist perspective?

7   IMPLICATIONS FOR

PRACTICE

Be Sure

If you want something real badly
And you're feeling insecure
There is only one thing I've got to tell you
And that is to be sure

Be positive
It's your prerogative
You're the only one who can open up the doors
Life is full of decisions
Make sure yours are not poor
(Christopher Richard Kwaku Kyem 1994)

Framework for anti-oppressive practice

We hope that by the end of Part I you had an understanding of the theories and ideologies informing anti-oppressive practice and the legislation which impinges on the work of health and welfare workers and carers. We do not for one minute suggest that this is easy or that you now have it all sorted out in your head. However, our intention was to provide the backdrop for Part II, where we went on to look at some of the elements we consider to be important in developing a model of anti-oppressive practice.

The model we now present will incorporate these elements into a clearer picture. By the end of this chapter you should have a framework which can be used in practice. This framework is informed by the preceding chapters and based on Phillipson's (1992) model of anti-oppressive practice. We have arrived at this modified version through our own experiences of working with people in various situations. You may wish to use this model, adapt it or develop your own – but we offer it as a first step.

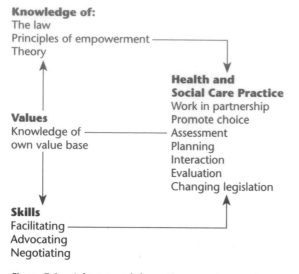

Knowledge of:
The law
Principles of empowerment
Theory

Values
Knowledge of
own value base

**Health and
Social Care Practice**
Work in partnership
Promote choice
Assessment
Planning
Interaction
Evaluation
Changing legislation

Skills
Facilitating
Advocating
Negotiating

Figure 7.1   A framework for anti-oppressive practice.

The model, shown diagrammatically in Figure 7.1, takes as given an acknowledgement of the reality of oppression and inequality that exists in society. The next stage is what impact that has on us. It is how we experience the reality of oppression (our biography) which determines our response and so inevitably shapes our *value* base. Our understanding of that reality then propels us to go and seek out the *knowledge* about the issues and information needed to develop *skills* which will combat oppression and inequality. This then leads on to the third stage, which is how our knowledge, values and skills are brought together in such a way that our care and practice with others is empowering at both the personal and structural levels.

The model is never static, in so far as we have constantly to evaluate critically what we are doing. This enables us to change our response as we continue to seek out knowledge and develop our skills. Lynn (1991) suggests that we need a system of self-evaluation to enable us to develop an anti-oppressive perspective. Since anti-oppressive practice is about change, we can only develop such a perspective if we have an in-built system for critical self-analysis. Lynn provides a number of self-assessment questions (which we have amended slightly to include carers) to assist in this process. We can assure you from our own experience that these questions are challenging and far from easy to answer!

1 What theories and values inform my caring practice?
2 What is the likely impact of my perspective on users or the person I care for?

In our interactions with others we respond differently depending on whether they are female, male, black, white, working class, middle class, old, young, gay, lesbian, heterosexual, disabled, able-bodied. They will also respond to the differences they perceive in us. Taking account of the complexity and tensions in the dynamics of the situation, you therefore also need to ask:

3 How do I respond to all these differences?
4 Do I have a system of constantly analysing difference?

Why is this important? Let us illustrate this with the following question: 'How can you address the fine detail of anti-oppressive practice when there is no toilet for disabled people in this building?' The fact that there was no toilet for disabled people *is* the fine detail of oppression. So another question you have to ask is:

5 What is my definition of oppression?
6 How does it inform my practice?
7 What power do I have to change practice?

These seven questions, Lynn suggests, are individual challenges. To work in isolation saps our energy and can be demoralizing. Therefore, perhaps the most important question of all is:

8 What is my support network?

As we grow and develop our answers change. It is therefore useful to keep a record of your answers – which will also of course assist you to monitor your development.

Applying the model

In order to apply the model we will analyse the case of Kate. Kate is a 30-year-old black woman with two children, Nancy aged five and Mary Ann aged seven. After the birth of Nancy, her mental health deteriorated. This resulted in her marriage breaking down. She subsequently found it increasingly difficult to cope with the girls on her own, so she moved in with her mother and father. Kate's father Tom is 72 and in poor health, so that her mother Ann (aged 60) finds herself spending more and more time looking after her husband's needs. Life sometimes gets a bit difficult for Ann, as Kate is often unable to cope with the demands of her children and retreats, leaving Ann to cope. Ann loves Nancy and Mary Ann and feels that it is nice for Tom to have the children around. She also worries about her daughter's health and tries to protect her as much as she can. When Ann is really fed up and needs someone to talk to she turns to her younger daughter, Suzie, whom she sees once a week.

Oppression

The starting point here is to consider the oppressions that we can identify for various members of the family. Some of these include consideration of issues around mental health, including: the impact of racism in the mental health field; gender, related to the caring role in relation to the children and

Tom, and to motherhood (both for Kate and Ann); and age and the loss of independence that can come as people get older, which for Tom could include loss of status within the family.

The issue of race and mental health is a complex one and there is much documented evidence about the negative experiences black people have encountered within health and social care services (Torkington 1991). Research has shown that black people are more likely to be given major tranquillizers than white people; are more likely to see junior or unqualified psychiatrists; are more likely to be hospitalized than treated in the community or as outpatients; are twice as likely to be the subject of a Mental Health Act 'section' and so be held in a hospital involuntarily; and more likely to be treated with ECT and to be given more 'shocks' (Webb and Tossell 1991: 136). There has been a failure by social care agencies to provide a service that meets the needs of black communities. For example, black elders are significantly under-represented in local authority service provision for older people (Webb and Tossell 1991).

The expectations on women to be involved in the care of either related children or other adults are far greater than on men (Hamner and Statham 1988). This is viewed as a marginalized activity (Webb and Tossell 1991) and a feature of unpaid caring is that women are left isolated with limited support from family or friends (Finch 1989).

The personal reality of oppression

Kate (mother)

I really feel like I need to go to hospital for help. But I'm terrified because I went once and the next thing I knew they'd got an order to make me stay in the hospital and it was really hard to get out. I think they thought I was mad. That's why I don't take the drugs they give me. I don't think they help me. Suzie gets annoyed with me for not taking them. All I wanted was help so I can be a good mum. I'd like to be like my own mum – she manages to cope with Nancy and Mary Ann, so I should be able to. I never really wanted kids, but now I've got them I feel I ought to be able to be a proper mother. I feel like a break – then I'd be able to cope. But I don't think the doctors understand this. I think they think that because I've got mum then everything is all right. I remember when I went last time the doctor who gave me the drugs said he didn't know why I worried about the kids because people like us are used to all living together anyway.

Mary Ann (daughter)

They're always talking about my mum and what's wrong with her. If they think I'm listening they send me out of the room. Or sometimes they stop talking when I come in – and I know they've been talking about her. I get really sad. I wish they would talk to me and tell me properly what is happening. I do understand. Sometimes I stay off school to be with my mum when she's sad. I have to pretend I don't feel well otherwise grandma gets cross.

Tom (grandfather)

I get so tired. I wish I could do more to help Ann. She never seems to stop. When I feel ill I tend to shout at the girls. They're good children and I love having them around. But sometimes I just want the two of us to be alone. Often Ann is too tired to talk to me any more. I wish that Kate would get help so that we could get our lives back together again.

Ann (grandmother)

Poor little Nancy and Mary Ann. I worry about what is going to happen to them – I won't be here for ever. And Tom suffers too, although I know he likes to have the children around. I've been talking to Suzie about what to do for the best. Suzie's worried about what is happening to me and her dad and thinks that Kate should have a place of her own. Suzie seems to think she can get lots of help off social services and the hospital. I'm not so sure myself – I've never asked for anything. I've worked and I've managed all my life. They won't give me something for nothing but Suzie tells me I'm wrong – she seems to know these things.

Suzie (sister)

Why should my family suffer like this? They have a right to services. Kate should be able to live on her own and if she had the right help I know she could. Mum could still see her every day but not have the worry of caring for her. No one at home seems to be able to do what they really want – they should all be able to have a choice at the very least.

What next?

It is clear from the individual stories that each person in the family has her or his own feelings and experiences of oppression. It is our job to listen to all those viewpoints. You may think that it is unlikely that all in the family will tell you their story. You are right. They will not, and if they do, it will take time. We therefore need to be aware of what might be happening for each individual and be aware of their stories as part of a wider structure. If we are committed to empowering people we must be aware of how we can use legislation to mobilize resources, however hard that might be, and use our skills to increase available choices.

We can see that the stories of the various people involved present a number of dilemmas, both for the family members themselves and for any professionals who might be involved with them. The stories can therefore be seen as issues about personal responsibility, structural disadvantage or legal duty (Jordan 1990).

If we read these stories, firstly, in terms of the moral obligations of the people involved we could pose the following questions.

- Should Kate be totally responsible for the care of her children?
- Should Kate consider her parents and look for her own accommodation?

- Should Ann be burdened with the care of her grandchildren when she has the responsibility to care for her husband?
- Should Tom expect his wife to care for him or should social services be providing assistance?
- Does Mary Ann have an obligation to attend school?

This is not an exhaustive list – you may well be able to think of more questions along the same lines.

Secondly, the same stories could be read in terms of the structural disadvantages faced by those involved. For example, racism structures the delivery of health and care services. Women are often left with the burden of caring. Often this is because of the unequal power relationships between men and women (Finch and Groves 1980; Dalley 1983; Ungerson 1993). If we accept the structural nature of inequality we could argue that there is very little that can be done unless it is through political campaigning.

Thirdly, the stories could be read from a liberal/bureaucratic perspective, focussing on legal duty, and attempts will be made to fit the 'needs' of the individual family members into available resources. If Kate refuses to take her medication and deteriorates further then she will be compulsorily detained under the mental health legislation. If Mary Ann and Nancy are assessed as 'at risk' then they could be accommodated by the local authority and the parental burden could be shared with the local authority – otherwise they remain Kate's responsibility. Tom can be offered day care and it is up to Ann to fit her needs around this. If either Tom or Ann is unhappy about day care arrangements then little more can be offered. The essence of this reading of the stories is that social care practitioners work within clear legal boundaries with finite resources.

We would add a fourth perspective. Taking account of everyone's needs we would use the legislation as a resource to ensure that the rights and choices of all those involved were respected. We would focus on their needs, and attempt not to fit their needs into available resources, but to ensure that resources are available to meet their needs. This may seem a little idealistic, but anti-oppressive practice is about moving towards the ideal – making changes to the existing order.

Let us go back to Kate's story. A social worker has been asked to visit the family after Suzie approaches the social services department with Ann. The social worker completes the assessment and makes the following observations.

- *Kate* wants to move into her own accommodation but is worried about how she will cope.
- *Mary Ann's* attendance at school has deteriorated over the past two months. She has strong attachments to both her mother and her grandparents.
- *Nancy* is quite clingy to her mother. She is very close to Mary Ann, who often gets her ready for school in the mornings. Like Mary Ann she likes living with her grandparents, but if Kate moved into her own home Nancy would like to be able to see her grandmother every day.
- *Tom* is mentally alert and fiercely independent. He sometimes needs help with daily care tasks. He misses meeting his friends at the local club.

- *Ann* finds all the care tasks tiring. She knows that Kate would like a place of her own but has never encouraged it as she's worried how she would cope on her own. Part of her would also miss having the children around. Sometimes she feels that so much of her time and energy is spent on Kate that her other daughter suffers, as the time spent with Suzie is usually taken up talking about Kate or the children. Ann feels that she rarely has time to ask Suzie about her own life.
- *Suzie* is worried about her parents and feels that they have aged a lot since Kate went to live with them. She thinks the social services, the hospital and their own medical practitioner are just not interested and so are failing to meet the needs of any of the family members.

The process of assessment

The family all recognize that to continue living under the same roof could become increasingly stressful and jeopardize the relationships they all currently enjoy. The social worker then works with Kate to link in with the community support networks to enable Kate to manage independently. She takes on the role of advocate for Kate with the housing department.

The social worker is aware that it is not necessary to be roofless to be classified as homeless (Housing Act 1985, Part III). Kate is not legally entitled to occupy her parent's accommodation and therefore can be defined as homeless. She could also be 'threatened' with homelessness by her parents if the situation became untenable. These were some of the arguments the social worker used in discussions with the housing department. This was a difficult battle, and required all her professional advocacy skills.

The first step was to get the housing authority to accept that Kate could be classified as homeless. Part of the social worker's argument in support of the application for accommodation was in terms of preventing the family from breaking down and safeguarding the welfare of the children. Here she drew on the Children Act 1989 by defining them as being 'in need', underpinned by the principles of the Act concerning keeping families together and working in partnership with other local authority departments.

The social worker then worked with Kate to link in with the community support networks to enable Kate to manage independently. She also spent some time talking to Mary Ann about her reluctance to go to school. Having identified some of the issues, she was able to work with Mary Ann towards an acceptable solution for everyone. This involved Mary Ann saying that she would talk to a particular teacher in the school when she was worried about her mother, rather than stay away from school. In this way the social worker was able to negotiate with Mary Ann an acceptable way of liaising with the school in offering her support without her being inappropriately 'labelled'. In this respect the social worker's practice is informed by the principles of legislation concerning the importance of involving young people in the decision making processes about their lives.

Having done this, the social worker considered the needs of Tom and Ann. Under Section 47 of the National Health Service and Community Care Act

1990 an assessment of need should be carried out. From this the social worker was able to work with them to decide how to meet those needs. She was mindful of the requirement under Section 20 of the Race Relations Act 1976 that decisions on providing services have to be non-discriminatory. Section 71 of the same Act also requires local authorities:

> to make appropriate arrangements with a view to securing that their various functions are carried out with due regard to the need –
> a) to eliminate unlawful racial discrimination; and
> b) to promote equality of opportunity and good relations, between persons of different racial groups.

So the social worker was prepared to argue her case for specific services to meet Tom's needs.

We have tried to illustrate briefly some of the possible ways of working in partnership with a family in a particular situation to resolve the dilemmas presented. Although we have only focused on the social worker, there are a number of health and social care practitioners who would be involved with the family. They should be working in partnership with the social worker and, equally importantly, should be aware of those elements of the law which could be harnessed to provide a successful outcome. The outcome presented here is by no means the only solution, but we intend it to be illustrative rather than directive.

Final thoughts

Anti-oppressive practice is not easy. When practitioners are busy, with limited resources and minimal support systems, it becomes even more difficult. The easier option for health and social care practitioners can then be to 'muddle through' (Jordan 1990) and do only what we are legally bound to do – *which could be very little!* Alternatively we could respond to pressures from other professionals, from the community or from family members (such as Suzie in the above example), forgetting the principles which should underpin our practice. Those pressures *could* direct us to using the law oppressively, reacting to situations of crisis. However, it *is* possible to use our knowledge of the law, our values and our skills (the basis of our framework for practice) in applying the law to work from an anti-oppressive perspective – to use legislation as a resource whereby we can provide services which allow user groups an element of choice.

Part III REFRAMING PRACTICE

IN RELATION TO

LEGISLATION

8   PREVENTIVE

WORK

An ounce of prevention is worth a pound of cure.

In considering the concept of prevention we are instantly faced with the question of what is to be prevented. Skidmore *et al.* (1991: 328) suggest that prevention is about 'keeping the vase intact, rather than trying to repair the broken pieces'; that is, instead of 'gluing together human parts that have been cracked, broken apart or splintered', prevention for us is about keeping human personalities and interrelationships operational. But it could be argued that legislation which is aimed at encouraging the market economy and competitive tendering is unlikely to promote an increase in preventive service provision. Keeping the vase intact is about preventive work at the personal level, but what about the structural level? Is part of preventive work about preventing discrimination? Is the major focus of probation and juvenile justice work crime prevention? The first part of this chapter will consider what we mean by prevention. The second part of the chapter will then go on to look at what attention it has received from policy makers and practitioners. Finally we will consider some preventive strategies with various user groups.

What are we preventing?

Health and social welfare practice has drawn on medical models in developing preventive strategies. Five levels of prevention are, for example:

- health promotion;
- specific protection;
- early diagnosis and treatment;

- disability limitation;
- rehabilitation (Skidmore *et al.* 1991).

Levels of prevention in public health have also been described as primary, secondary and tertiary. In social care practice, the primary level is the 'health promotion' level: working positively with people to protect them for future 'good health'. The secondary level is about early diagnosis and treatment: relieving distress and reducing symptoms. At the tertiary level prevention tends to be more therapeutic and to enhance quality of life. Similar levels have been used in some local authority children's plans. One plan we have looked at describes four identified levels of family support.

1 *Prevention or 'diversion'*, which is targeted at welfare institutions, community networks and social policy. The dominant mode of practice at this level is community action, community development and community social work.
2 *'Early prevention'*, which is targeted at family systems, support networks and welfare institutions. The dominant mode of practice is generic, multi-role practitioner, social care planning and social casework.
3 *'Heavy-end' prevention*, which is targeted at personal change, with the dominant mode of practice being individual casework and treatment or therapy.
4 *Intervention or 'early restoration'*, which is targeted at personal change, with the objectives of intervention being to secure the welfare of the child, to reduce risks to the child and to reduce conflicts with the child (e.g. within the family, with the criminal law); the dominant mode of practice is treatment or therapy (Metropolitan Borough of Stockport Children's Services Division 1994/5).

If we consider prevention in child care practice we can see that historically it refers to anything from abuse and neglect, admission to care, court appearances for young offenders, provision of nursery places to child minding and so on. More recently it has been underpinned by the value system which accompanies the ideology of the family and consequently state support for the family (Hardiker *et al.* 1989). If one reads the children's plans produced by social services departments they all, as they are indeed required to do, indicate policy plans for preventive services. However, the Children Act 1989 also lays a legal duty on all agencies to work together. This means that a wider definition of preventive work is written into some documents. For example, Rochdale Children's Plan 1993 considers specific targets for children and young people as identified in *Health of the Nation*, which sets targets for health authorities and family health services authorities:

- To reduce the suicide rate of people (including young people) with mental health problems by at least 33 per cent by the year 2000.
- To reduce by at least 50 per cent the rate of conception among the under 16s by the year 2000.
- To reduce the death rate from accidents among those under 15 by 33 per cent and among those aged from 15 to 24 years by 25 per cent by the year 2005.

In terms of health promotion it includes a commitment to encourage people, especially young people, to stop smoking and to drink less alcohol.

In considering why preventive work is such a difficult issue we have to think about the impact of complex social policies, inadequate resources and changing attitudes. If we take a look at the last of these we can see that much child care practice, for instance, focuses on child protection rather than on looking at the needs of children. This may remove some oppressed and vulnerable families from the arena for preventive and supporting services.

There is also the problem of prioritizing not only within various user groups but also between them. Policies of prevention and health care mean that people are living longer and enjoy better health. However, the likelihood is that in the end they will become more dependent and therefore increase the calls on resources. And then, the question could be asked, who should the housing department consider a priority when a transfer to a ground floor flat becomes available: the lone parent with small children or the older person who finds difficulty with stairs or lift?

Preventive work with older people raises a lot of other questions. Again we have to ask what is the object of prevention for older people (Tinker 1981). It cannot be avoidance of death because that is inevitable. It may be possible to prevent expensive forms of care if preventive measures are introduced early enough. Or it may be that preventing an accident or entry into institutional care can save money and human suffering. Government guidelines have stated that prevention is the key to healthier living and a higher quality of life for everyone. So, for example, chiropody services and greater attention to feet can prevent older people being unnecessarily housebound. Equally, adequate dental care, eye care and attention to hearing can only assist in maintaining older people within the community. The role of health visitors and occupational therapists is vital in this respect, to provide support in the community and arrange aids and adaptations. Again this indicates how the principles of partnership between agencies are never more important than in preventive work.

Generally speaking it can be argued that preventive work is necessary to prevent the need for more intrusive alternatives in the long term. In many ways it could be said that preventive work is the most empowering form of health and social care practice. So what are we required to do by law? And how can we use the legislation to maximize the development of preventive strategies?

What are our duties and responsibilities?

Preventive work has to be understood in relation to social policies. Social policy under Conservative governments has been based on the political philosophy of the nineteenth century: so strategies have been based on residual and selective services rather than universal; there is an emphasis on the mixed economy of welfare already mentioned, and the centrality of the family as key providers of care and units of social responsibility (Tunstil 1989).

Briefly, to understand social policies we can look at the models of welfare which underpin them.

1 *Residual model.* Care of children is not the business of the state. Individuals and families carry the burden of responsibility to provide for all needs. The state intervenes as a last resort, and only to provide a *basic social minimum* if parenting leads to a level of care which threatens the well-being of a child (or other client group). Within this model social care practitioners are agents of social control.

2 *Institutional model.* The role of the state is to meet the needs of the most disadvantaged members of society. It does this through coordination of the mixed market economy. Social care practitioners assess needs and provide services to address them. It has been said to be 'a more humane method of social control' (Hardiker *et al.* 1989), which aims at social integration (rather than, for example, rescuing children and punishing parents).

3 *Developmental model.* Here there is a greater role for the state as a means towards a more just and equal society. Social problems are not the sole responsibility of individuals and families, nor a consequence of inefficient service delivery, but are products of deep-rooted social inequalities. The state accepts responsibility to meet needs through universal social services and redistributive social policies. Social care practitioners are agents of change – empowerment, mediation, advocacy and community participation are used to facilitate this.

Health and social welfare agencies offer minimalist residual services and resources are aimed at families most 'at risk'. In a political and social climate where material and social resources for families are declining, health and social care practitioners and carers have to make every effort to address themselves to political and social realities in order to achieve positive preventive services.

On a more general level preventive work could be seen to be enshrined in the concept of equality. This is a complex area but, for example, it could mean *equality of access* to a living income (we cannot direct the wealth or income processes of society but we can enable equality of access). Often people who use social care services are disadvantaged in the job market, or indeed are excluded from it – for example, because they are disabled. The role of practitioners and carers might then be to seek for improved access to work opportunities. One could also consider *equality of social integration* – this of course is considered in the community care legislation in terms of expanding and improving community care services, including the preventive functions, improving the quality of residential care and delabelling stigmatizing conditions. Finally there is *equality of power* – by empowering users and giving them the opportunity to control service provision, by working in partnership and encouraging participation.

Strategies for action

Here we present some strategies for action and examples of preventive work with different user groups.

Safe houses

If a young person is considering the choices and options available to resolve a particular problem it could well be that the preferred option is to run away. Indeed this could, on occasions, be the least detrimental alternative.

> Janice was terrified of her father. When he was drunk he would hit her and when he was sober he would ridicule her. She was frightened to tell anyone in case they didn't believe her. She was convinced that life would get worse if he found out that she had told anyone. So she ran away.

Running away is often the only way young people can be heard. Research from the Central London Teenage Project (CLTP) indicates the importance of providing somewhere for young runaways. While it may be hard immediately to see how this fits into the category of preventive work, one of the social workers interviewed in the research believed that safe houses not only empowered young people in care but also gave them the opportunity to talk to professionals who would work with them to negotiate possible alternatives.

Perhaps one of the most important aspects of the research was that the safe house gave the young people the opportunity to take stock. It identified the importance of addressing the reasons why young people run away if their situation is to be resolved. It demonstrated the need for resources to give young people ongoing support on their return to their homes or care placements. So safe houses can prevent further incidents of running away. They also provide shelter, care and a place of safety – this last being vital since in order to support themselves some young people 'who had found themselves hungry, penniless and with no place to go had turned to prostitution' which of course means that they 'risked both their health and their lives' (Newman 1989: 142). Other positive comments from social workers indicated that safe houses can give workers a 'lever to push for action' or empower young people by giving them a bargaining position.

Section 51 of the Children Act 1989 recognizes the need for refuges for young people at risk and gives the Secretary of State power to issue certificates with respect to voluntary or registered homes or foster carers approved by local authorities or voluntary organizations. Children and young people can be taken into and remain in a refuge if they appear to be at risk of harm (Reg. 3(2) The Refuges (Children's Homes and Foster Placements) Regulations 1991). There are limitations placed on the length of time a young person may stay in a refuge (Reg. 3(9)), but if the people running the refuge feel that leaving would cause significant harm there are options available to safeguard that young person (Section 46, Police Protection; Section 44(1), Emergency Protection Order). The guidance acknowledges the need for safe houses when it states that

> Refuge workers can work with the youngsters to help them to return to parents or local authority care, or to sort out some other solution if a return home is not appropriate (e.g. where a child has been, or may have been, sexually or physically or emotionally abused at home).
>
> (DoH 1991c: 4, para. 9.4)

Protecting women and children in violent situations

One could argue that for women trying to escape from situations of domestic violence we must be talking about gluing the vase back together rather than keeping it intact. However, it is important to give some consideration to the matter under the heading of prevention, particularly if one defines preventive work as preventing the need for more intrusive intervention. In the case of domestic violence more intrusive intervention could occur in relation to child protection. Links between domestic violence and child abuse are now being recognized (Merchant 1993). Social services departments have no statutory responsibility to protect women, and 'the law is a blunt instrument in protecting a person from domestic violence' (Brayne and Martin 1990: 287). However, social services departments do have a statutory responsibility to protect children and to help women to protect their children.

It has been suggested that the basic principle for good practice must be that the protection and empowerment of women is the most effective form of child protection (Merchant 1993). If a woman is worried about leaving her home because of very real fears about money and a roof over her head then practitioners need to know how to apply to a court for maintenance for the woman (if she is married) and to the Child Support Agency for the children. Equally, workers need to be aware that a woman cannot be treated as intentionally homeless under the Housing Act 1985 if she leaves a violent situation. It is further suggested in the code of guidance that to leave because of threatened violence is also not considered to be deliberate.

While domestic violence is not mentioned in the Children Act 1989, the Women's Aid Federation England has pointed out that children who are in refuges as a result of domestic violence are children 'in need' and as such qualify for all the support and preventive services of any child defined as 'in need'. The Children Act Advisory Committee has recognized that protecting children within the home where there is domestic violence is limited. 'The Committee considers that the law and procedure in this area does not adequately assist in protecting the welfare of children' (Annual Report 1992/3: 22). In situations where the parents are married a court may make an order excluding a spouse from the matrimonial home 'if a child of the family is in danger of being physically injured by the respondent' under the Domestic Proceedings and Magistrates' Courts Act 1978, but there are a lot of limitations as to when an exclusion order might be made.

Prevention in such cases means ensuring that what Liz Kelly of the Child Abuse Studies Unit at the University of North London has indicated may be 'far reaching consequences of the abuse and their mother's struggles to end it' (Marchant 1993: 7) do not result in long-term intervention by social care agencies. The legal implications of the woman's situation may well be complex and it therefore requires not only a knowledge of the legal provisions about domestic violence but also an understanding of the 'complexity and variety of legal knowledge' that can apply in such situations (Vernon 1993: 104).

Elder abuse

We discussed earlier in the chapter the fact that preventive medicine means that people are living longer. But this brings with it the problems of caring for frail older people. Abuse of older people has become more prominent as increasingly older people are staying in their own homes or being cared for by relatives. In May 1993 *Community Care* launched a campaign called 'Elder abuse – break the silence' to alert people to the oppression of older people. While the Community Care Act (1990) recognizes the need to support and empower carers there is also a need to ensure that those being cared for are empowered. One of the most interesting aspects of this campaign was the fact that it highlighted ways of using existing legislation while also pushing the government to produce guidelines and linking in to the Law Commission's proposals for statutory powers. A brief look at some of the issues will demonstrate how existing legislation could be used to prevent elder abuse while one is working at a structural level towards a situation where 'the bandwagon of legislative change looks unstoppable' (Murray 1993: 16).

In launching the campaign, Eastman (1993a: 20) considered the problems of defining elder abuse. In his exploration of the dilemmas he argued that there were four principles to bear in mind:

- abuse is wrong and a criminal offence;
- a definition should make its moral base explicit and be owned by the agency;
- carers have power over dependent vulnerable relatives regardless of the stresses of caring;
- a definition should help with the confrontation and reduce the numbers of older people at risk, as otherwise the definition is meaningless.

To reflect the fact that abuse is unlawful he considered the police definitions of abuse. Such definitions may not take in the stresses faced by carers. However, they are helpful in reminding us that when no legal powers exist to intervene in cases of suspected elder abuse there are other ways of considering a situation. Police definitions of abuse are as follows.

- Common assault: pushing, thumping, forced medication, pulling hair.
- Actual bodily harm: physical sign of assault including emotional/psychological abuse.
- Grievous bodily harm (with intent).
- Manslaughter.
- Murder.
- Theft: dishonestly appropriating property belonging to another with the intention of permanently depriving the owner of it.

Such definitions immediately make things clearer, even if it is still not easy to detect abuse. One area that is particularly difficult, however, is that of financial abuse.

Research by Teri Whittaker (1993), lecturer in community care at Liverpool University, shows that financial abuse is the most common form of abuse. Debates are ongoing about the adequacy of the law to protect older people from financial abuse. While an older person can give someone *power of attorney* and the Court of Protection can assist the financial affairs of those who suffer from a mental disorder, there are many who feel that legal changes should be made to protect older people still further. However, Whittaker feels that the available legislation is sufficient and that what is needed is for professionals to be more aware of how to use it. She argues that professionals should use their personal power to prevent financial abuse by talking to relatives.

While, then, it can be argued that legislation does exist for preventing financial abuse, it is perhaps less easy to prevent emotional abuse. Mervyn Eastman's model, however, shows that it can be placed within the police category of actual bodily harm. He explains:

> My sense of emotional abuse is that it is actual and it is real, as opposed to the argument that discounts it in relation to physical abuse. I feel that any behaviour by a person in a position of power, which has a consequence for the other person – such as being tearful, incontinent or depressed – is emotional abuse.
>
> (Eastman 1993b: 18)

It may often be health care professionals and hospital social workers who will become aware of emotional abuse through assessment. Since assessments for care packages are written into the legislation it is incumbent on those undertaking the assessments and psychogeriatricians to be aware of the indicators that an older person is being emotionally abused.

Often those who do the assessments are social workers and it could be that older people would accept help from a district nurse but not from a social worker (Cohen 1993). It is important, therefore, for health and social care practitioners to work together with each other (as well as with carers and service users) in order to make informed assessments. In particular, the role of general practitioners is vital. Before any decision to provide nursing care is made a medical practitioner must be consulted (Section 55, NHSCCA). There is also the contract for general practitioners to screen all those over 74 years of age. Obviously it is no easier to detect elder abuse than it is abuse of children and young people. What the legislation provides, though, is the opportunity to assess the needs of people rather than just provide a service. This must provide the opportunity to be more aware of possible elder abuse for those referred for assessment, particularly if local authorities have guidelines about elder abuse to go with the assessment procedure.

The legislation also offers better choice of residential or nursing care for older people. This should then make it more possible for an older person to leave an abusive situation. The opportunities are there – workers need to empower themselves to recognize and confront elder abuse, however, if preventive strategies are to be developed.

Finally, the legislation does also give local authorities the opportunity to provide carers with support. While Eastman has argued that carers have been empowered at the expense of older people, who need to be equally empowered, it is important to remember that carers also need a tremendous amount of support. This means more than just recognizing the stresses of caring – it means recognizing the family dynamics and multiple problems that families experience, such as mental illness or problem drinking. While it has been pointed out that the legislation could be unconsciously sustaining abuse where the carer is the perpetrator (Cohen 1993), that should not be used as a justification for rationing resources.

Crime prevention

It has been suggested that social service departments generally and juvenile justice teams in particular should 'make an appropriate contribution to crime prevention strategies' (NACRO 1991: 1). Equally, one of the objectives of probation orders is to prevent the offender from committing further offences. To illustrate the point we will briefly look at some of the issues in relation to juvenile crime.

Frost and Stein (1989) refer to *structural* crime prevention as the starting point for a progressive agenda for responding to juvenile crime. This has three dimensions:

1 Macro-economic, distributional and employment strategies to challenge the oppression of young people.
2 The development of educational, youth and community and recreational services which are characterized by the development of anti-discriminatory practice strategies.
3 *Situational* crime prevention aimed at inner-city environmental regeneration.

NACRO (1991) recognizes the central role of juvenile justice workers in developing youth crime prevention strategies, as well as their primary role in reducing the numbers of young people going to court and into custody. In this respect, Schedule 7 of the Children Act 1989 lays a *duty* on local authorities to 'take reasonable steps designed . . . to encourage children within their area not to commit criminal offences'. Department of Health guidance stresses the obligations of local authorities to prevent juvenile crime. Thus, NACRO points out, just as the Act requires a different approach to child care work it also requires different ways of working for juvenile justice workers to prevent the involvement of young people in crime. Such an approach should use the lessons learned from the development of diversionary approaches in juvenile justice and 'a social crime prevention approach which aims to improve the quality of life for all young people who are disadvantaged' (NACRO 1991: 3). A central feature of such strategies would acknowledge and challenge social divisions (Frost and Stein 1989).

Discrimination

As we indicated in Part I, anti-discriminatory practice must be a part of anti-oppressive practice. Many groups of people face intense discrimination in various areas of their lives. It is therefore essential that social care practitioners are aware of the reality of users' lives in order to practise from an empowerment perspective at both the personal and the structural levels. It is also necessary to be aware of case law that is pertinent to specific situations, to lobby about unfair discrimination and to ensure that wherever we are working there are clear policy statements regarding anti-discriminatory practice. In order to illustrate these points we will briefly consider three particular groups of people, although the issues raised have implications for work in any situation where a person or group of people suffers discrimination.

Disabled persons

The reality of the lives of disabled people is that they are often barred from many leisure activities or from using public transport, and are discriminated against in employment (Oliver 1991; Morris 1993a). They often find themselves in poverty not only as a result of unemployment but also because they have to pay more for services such as transport, since they are denied access to the cheaper forms of public transport. Employment opportunities are further limited by the inaccessibility of buildings and transport. Even enlightened local authorities with clear equal opportunity statements often have municipal buildings which are inaccessible and support inadequate public transport systems.

It could be argued that legislation does exist to assist disabled people in employment because companies with more than 20 staff are required to employ disabled people as 3 per cent of their staff. However, not only is this often ignored but also it stigmatizes disabled people. Many disabled people feel that the assumption is that they are inferior and that they are not necessarily employed on merit but because there is a compulsion for them to be given a job. Nevertheless, it does provide some legal form of redress for disabled people.

In an attempt to provide more adequate legal safeguards for disabled people the Disabled Persons (Civil Rights) Bill was brought before Parliament in 1993. Unfortunately, although it attracted widespread media debate and vigorous debate in Parliament, like previous Bills on the same subject it was ignored by those in power. At the level of action, therefore, practitioners need to work with disabled people to ensure that the lobby for anti-discriminatory legislation remains on the agenda. At the same time, health and social care practitioners and carers need to lobby within their own environments to prevent discrimination against disabled people.

Travellers

The reality of life for travellers is that discrimination is so acute that at both individual and collective levels they face insecurity and harsh living conditions and are denied access to social, educational and health services (Pahl and Vaile 1986). They argue that the problem has been 'one of the criminalisation of Gypsies through institutionalised racism' (Northern Gypsy Council 1992: 2). In the past travellers' contact with social services has led to children being separated from their families and culture through the care system.

The Children Act 1989, however, offers the opportunity for practitioners to consider the context of the lives of travellers and to work from an anti-oppressive perspective to promote change and lessen the inequalities of their lives (King 1988; Cemlyn 1993).

At both an individual and a collective level the principles underpinning the legislation – such as partnership, minimal intervention, parental responsibility, consideration of racial and cultural background, consideration of the wishes and feelings of children and their parents, provisions relating to children defined as 'in need' and duties in relation to homeless young people – enable practitioners to work with travellers in a positive way. By way of illustration there are two aspects of the legislation which can be particularly helpful in this respect. First, the need to consider the religious, racial, cultural and linguistic background of children is particularly important. This can validate the way of life for travellers. Secondly, the definition of need in Section 17 of the Children Act 1989 means that some traveller children become eligible for its provisions because of the living conditions that they have to endure as a result of poor amenities provided by local authorities.

Young lesbians and gay men

The reality of the lives of young lesbians and gay men, particularly those looked after by social care agencies, is that:

- being lesbian or gay is wrong and they should be referred for treatment;
- they have to prove that they are 'really gay';
- those adults who are sympathetic find it difficult to support young lesbian or gay people as they are afraid of being labelled themselves.

The problem is most acute in faith-based voluntary agencies which provide services for young people. However, both statutory and voluntary agencies fail fully to address the problem. This is not made any easier by the existence of Clause 28. It could be argued that one way of assisting young lesbians and gay men is by allocating lesbian or gay workers. Clearly their own experiences of oppression can only help a young person in a similar situation. However, workers can find it difficult as they encounter prejudice and stereotyped views among colleagues, and have to work within a legal framework where the 'promotion' of homosexuality is illegal. However, the Children Act 1989 does recognize that 'Gay young men and women may require very sympathetic carers to enable them to accept their sexuality and to develop their own self esteem' (DoH 1991c: 4, para. 9.53).

It is important, if discrimination against young lesbians and gay men is to be eradicated – despite the discriminatory legislation – for practitioners and carers to use the positive elements of legislation which exist, to discuss sexuality with young people, to ensure that their wishes and feelings are heard and that decisions are made in their best interests. Although guidance is only considered as secondary legislation, practitioners and carers must use whatever elements of policy, guidance and statute they can in order to develop preventive practice strategies in this area.

Final thoughts

> The logic of prevention suggests that resources should be focused on potentially successful situations where by putting in resources at an earlier stage, the point of collapse is not reached.
>
> (Twigg and Atkin 1994: 149)

Prevention requires creative thinking and imaginative use of resources. The prevention argument assumes, of course, that collapse can be avoided, or that it is possible to keep the vase intact. Realistically, one of the challenges for health and social care practitioners is how personal, family and community problems can be prevented. This means being aware of inequalities, and particularly of how to use what legislative frameworks are available, to prevent further discrimination against vulnerable groups of people.

One of the most important roles that practitioners have to play in prevention is that of networking. An essential element of anti-oppressive practice is that practitioners should not be working in isolation. 'Making and maintaining links between organisations and between individuals involved in caring and the organisations that might help (or hinder) them is a vital part of social care' (Payne 1993: 1). By sharing resources and making links organizations can work together to develop preventive strategies. Networking enables health and social care service providers to identify gaps and barriers. This then enables inter-agency collaboration in planning services to address unmet needs. Recent legislation envisages such collaboration as an essential aspect of health and social care practice, which in itself brings together many aspects of anti-oppressive practice.

Activity

The following exercise will enable you to assess the aims of the links that you currently make with other organizations. From this, you should be able to identify – in terms of your networking – whether you are constantly working in a reactive way, or are developing proactive strategies which will promote preventive ways of working.

The aims that may be fulfilled by making links can be divided into service, maintenance and policy aims. *Service aims* are concerned with providing effective services to the public. An essential aspect of linking which meets the aims of your service might be good practical relationships with agencies that refer potential users of the service, accept referrals from you or assist users. *Maintenance aims* are about keeping the agency in being so that the service aims can be met, e.g. regular contact with funding bodies and the support of other departments or councillors, if the service is a local authority one. *Policy aims* are concerned with changing policies which affect the service users in your area – these can be policies in other organizations and departments, or in government.

1 List all the links with other organizations that you have, and should have.
2 In each case decide whether the link meets service aims, maintenance aims or policy aims, or a combination of these, and the reason why it meets those aims.

3 For each list (service, maintenance, policy) rank the organization in order of priority for meeting that aim (i.e. top priority = 1, next priority = 2, etc.).
4 For each organization, add up the number given under each list to give the priority for linkages for that organization overall (the lower the number, the higher the priority).
5 If you are working alone look at each priority ranking, and consider whether it fits with your judgement of the priority. Are there factors which give it a higher or lower priority in the exercise which you are not thinking of in your work? If you are working with others, try sharing your judgements and testing with colleagues the reasons for them. If you are working on a team's links, how do your judgements agree? Are there significant differences in priority? How could you handle this (e.g. by each member taking on links that he or she personally gives high priority to)? Should you be trying to agree priorities? (From Payne 1993: 16.)

9 ASSESSMENT

Why do they write things about me?
Details of everything I do.
Why do they always watch me?
Wherever I may go.
Why do they make me stay in?
And if I go out, it's with them.
Why do they send me a counsellor
To find out things about me?
Why do they watch how I react
To problems we face each day?
Why do they assess me
When I have the right to be free?
Why do they label me –
When I am only being me!

(Chrissie Elms Bennett 1994)

What is assessment?

In discussing the term 'assessment', Zarb (1991: 197) suggests that it is a term that is 'clearly ideologically loaded'. He suggests, in relation to the needs of people who are ageing with a disability, that assessment reflects the power relationships between professionals and disabled people. This means that it is the *professionals* who define and assess the needs, rather than allowing disabled people to define their own needs. He argues, therefore, that people with disabilities are unable to retain control over how they may wish to live, their options are limited by the process and thus they are denied their legitimate rights. This creates an enforced dependency on providers to meet their needs. More practically, he states that the inflexibility of this professionally controlled assessment leads directly to the provision of inappropriate and wasteful services.

One way of overcoming the inflexibility of assessment processes has been the development of self-assessment. Morris (1993a) argues that if disabled people are to resist such inflexible assessments then they must be allowed to state clearly what are their own defined needs. This will enable them to counter the political nature of assessments which are used to distribute limited resources (Cornwell 1992). Perhaps more accurately, self-assessment is about involvement of the user in the process. This process is one 'in which the real feelings, needs and wishes of the individual can be discovered' (Hepinstall 1992).

However, there are many situations where, legally, social care practitioners are expected to assess. These are multiple and complex, and can be controversial. Some appear to be more oppressive, as in assessment of the need to use compulsory powers for instance, and some assist in the professional task. This is not to imply that the use of compulsory powers is of itself oppressive. However, the use of compulsion raises issues about social control and 'questions about the nature of the relationship between worker and client, about power, influence, persuasion and coercion' (Stevenson 1989: 157). Oppression involves abusing power, rather than using it. But the assessment can result in action which appears to be oppressive, since even if the motive is protection, 'to remove any person from their home against their will is considered to be one of the most extreme forms of coercion' (Stevenson 1989: 156). In opposition to Zarb's argument, therefore, it has been suggested that the nature of assessment is such that it is appropriate for experts with professional knowledge and judgement to be used as the central resource in the assessment of client situations (Kopp 1989).

Whichever point of view one takes, assessment cannot and does not take place without being affected by the attitudes and values of the assessor as well as the situation of the person(s) being assessed. 'Ideally, the assessment should be a forum in which hypotheses are devised and theories tested; a place where conflicting ideas are encouraged. The totally "objective" assessment remains an elusive ideal' (Pitts 1990: 54). If we endeavour to ensure that the assessment process incorporates the views of those being assessed then we are able to challenge 'professional assumptions of what need is and how it should be met' (Morris 1993a: 175).

In this chapter we will consider some of the dilemmas faced by practitioners, carers and service users in legislating for assessment. We will do this by considering specific issues within various pieces of legislation before providing a framework for anti-oppressive assessment.

Assessment is not value free

In the *Care Management and Assessment: Practitioners' Guide* published by the Department of Health Social Services Inspectorate (1991b) it is stated that care management and assessment lies at the heart of community care legislation. The guide recognizes that needs are unique to the individual concerned and these needs have to be identified and addressed but met within the available resources. It emphasizes a needs-led approach and that services should be more responsive. The Children Act 1989 also introduces the concept of need and Part III of that Act is devoted to outlining the provision of services for children defined as 'in need'.

Assessment of need is also about allocation of resources. Resources are limited, so assessment of need has been written into the legislation, in order to facilitate the distribution of resources. The concept of need presupposes that:

• we have a common understanding of what human need is;
• some needs are more deserving of resources than others;
• need is based on everyone being able to compete equally within society and to reach her or his full potential;
• need is based on maintaining a quality of life that enables us to participate in society;
• we can accurately assess need and provide the resources to meet it.

Assessment of need has to take into account the social dimension of people's lives. For example, the needs of a gay man, a black woman, a young person with a disability and an older person living alone will be very different and can really only be clearly defined by themselves.

The guidance accepts that need is a complex concept. It defines need in terms of 'the requirements of individuals to enable them to achieve, maintain or restore an acceptable level of social independence or quality of life, as defined by the particular care agency or authority' (DoH 1991b: 12). Clearly the notions of partnership and choice are severely limited by this definition. While one can recognize resource constraints, and even the need to allocate resources fairly, it seems a little incongruous that officials are defining 'quality of life' while there is increasing emphasis on the role of users and carers in the process (Stevenson and Parsloe 1993). Indeed, it has been noted that the government has never considered the idea that people should be involved in the assessment of their own needs (Walker 1991).

This point can be illustrated by a consideration of the legislation for people with disabilities. Guidance on developing assessment procedures placed emphasis on enabling people to 'live a full life in the community' and to 'be in charge of their own lives and make their own decisions, including decisions to take risks' (DoH 1991b). Disabled people do have the right under the 1986 Disabled Persons Act to ask for a comprehensive assessment of their needs. Local authorities also have a duty to provide services under Section 2 of the 1970 Chronically Sick and Disabled Persons Act. Resource problems cannot be used as a reason for not providing services. A genuine needs-led assessment incorporates the self-defined needs of disabled people. An anti-oppressive perspective would ensure that self-assessment and advocacy services are an essential element of community care policies, which then promote the rights of users (Morris 1993a).

Let us look at the experiences of Mark Hazell and his family. This case provides us with knowledge which could be used to enable us to improve our practice. The situation shows how practice can be needs-led rather than service-led. In July 1993 Mark Hazell won a court battle to live in the home he had chosen. Avon Social Services, in working from a service-led philosophy within certain financial constraints, was deemed to have failed in its attempts to meet Mark's needs.

Mark was a young man with learning difficulties, but, like anyone else his age, wanted to leave his family home. In order to do this he needed the help of Avon Social Services. To find an appropriate long-term placement an assessment of Mark's needs was necessary. However, the council's view of his needs conflicted with that of Mark and his family. Avon Social Services assessed that they could be met in an establishment that was considerably cheaper than the one preferred by Mark. It was this, rather than Mark's needs, that appeared to determine the decision. This conflict in opinion led Mark and his family to use the process of the law through judicial review to ensure that Mark's needs were met.

This case reminds us of the need to ensure that others in similar positions have access to information, support and guidance about the use of the law, so that their rights are not violated.

Children Act: minimal delay

In Section 1 of the Children Act 1989, one of the principles concerning the welfare of the child is the avoidance of delay (Section 1(2)) which creates uncertainty and has an impact on the relationship between children and their parents (Guidance and Regulations Volume 1, para. 1.8). The court is therefore required to draw up a timetable (Sections 11, 32) and ensure that delay is minimal. It has been pointed out, though, that the Act does not say that delay is necessarily prejudicial but that it is 'likely' to prejudice welfare. Therefore workers should not be constrained by this principle (Freeman 1992).

There are some assessments which, it has been acknowledged, will need a longer period of time than the 12-week guideline (Children Act Advisory Committee 1992/3), e.g. psychiatric assessment of the child's relationship with the family or a residential assessment of the family's parenting abilities. An interim care order can be used to assist in the assessment process if workers are still in the process of gathering information to inform the decision making. In the case of *Re A (a Minor) (Care Proceedings)* [1993] 1 FCR 164, FD, it was felt appropriate to protect the child by the use of an interim care order while the assessment was completed. However, an interim care order should not be used for review purposes (*Re CN (a Minor) Care Order* [1992] 2 FCR 401, FD). There is also the facility to go back to the court to devise a new timetable, both to minimize delay and to explain why delay might be necessary. What about delay in bringing a case to court? The principle which informs the court process must also inform our practice in assessing need. Let us look at this principle in a practice example.

Lekha was a single parent who had been brought up in the care of the local authority. She had two young children whom she cared for with assistance and support from her social worker and health visitor. At the birth of her third child the two older children were fostered, since Lekha felt that she would be unable to cope with the other two as well as the baby on her own. The foster carer developed a good working relationship with Lekha. The two children, who were very close to their mother, felt secure. The family was reunited when the baby was four months old and Lekha felt that she would be able to manage. However, after a month she was struggling and the older children went back to the carer. Over the next two years the children went backwards and forwards between the mother and the carer.

The social services department was committed to working in partnership with Lekha and did this very well. However, the children became increasingly distressed and throughout the process it became clear that no one was looking at what was happening to the children; the partnership focused on the needs of the mother. At a planning meeting a discussion took place regarding the taking of care proceedings. It was concluded, however, that since the partnership with Lekha had not broken down there were insufficient grounds for legal action.

The foster carer pointed out that the children needed the security of an order for their welfare, and did not consider that this would damage the excellent partnership that she, or the local authority, had with Lekha. Nor did she feel that it would damage Lekha's relationship with her children – it was a case of sharing the care, since assessment had clearly identified that the capacity of Lekha to change was limited.

Let us look at some of the assumptions here: about the 'no order' principle and working in partnership. A Social Services Inspectorate (SSI 1992) study and departmental discussions with various local authorities found that there was a belief that the 'no order' principle meant that authorities had to demonstrate that partnership had broken down before an order could be made. The making of an order should not impede the process of partnership. It has been said that 'the two processes are not mutually exclusive' (Children Act Advisory Committee 1992/3: para. 2.21). This is evidenced in *Re D (Care Proceedings: Appropriate Order)* [1993] 2 FCR 88, FD.

This case emphasized the protection of a child by means of a care order, which is not incompatible with cooperation between parents and social services (Children Act Advisory Committee 1992/3). In Lekha's case failure of the social services to take action effectively resulted in 'secondary abuse' of the children, who suffered increasing harm by the delay in the taking of appropriate legal action.

To summarize, practitioners must be able to differentiate *purposeful delay* from *drift* (Children Act Advisory Committee 1992/3). Assessments should be ongoing. The arguments that an assessment cannot or should not be *rushed* and is incompatible with the principle of minimal delay do not really hold water. In some instances an assessment of a risk situation has to be made within tight time constraints. In practice it is not impossible to complete an initial assessment in a short space of time.

Mental health: legalized assault?

Mental health law poses a number of problems, particularly where assessment of need may also lead to deprivation of liberty.

Councillor Davies has been contacted by a number of Bill Valentine's neighbours, who are concerned because they are aware that on occasions he leaves the gas on. Bill regularly complains that the person from the home care service is stealing from him. Bill Valentine lives alone following the death of his wife last year. His daughter has noticed over a period of time that his behaviour became increasingly bizarre and recently contacted the medical practitioner, who subsequently called in a specialist. Bill was then admitted to hospital for assessment. He was persuaded to go 'voluntarily' although the use of compulsory powers under the Mental Health or the National Assistance Acts was considered. As a result of his admission he was diagnosed as having multi-infarct dementia.

The factors that led to Bill becoming a service user can be identified from the discussions that took place between the various people involved. They went something like this:

Cllr Davies: From what I've heard Bill is a real danger to everyone in that block of flats. It's in everyone's interests, including Bill's, that he should be taken into hospital.

Social worker: Well, our goal is to try and help Mr Valentine stay in the community. We are providing services and I obviously need to assess what else is needed.

Daughter: My dad has always said he wants to be able to stay at home and look after himself, ever since mum died. I respect that and want him to keep his dignity and his independence.

Cllr Davies: Well, from the reports I've heard there's not that much dignity in his life anyway. He should be forced to leave home and be cared for properly if he won't go on his own. Is it dignified for a frail old man to be left at such risk to himself and others?

Social worker: I personally am totally opposed to any talk of depriving him of his liberty in this way. To remove someone against his will is a very drastic step.

GP: Well, my position is clear. He needs medical attention, and we have a duty to ensure that he receives it. If that means that he has to be removed, then so be it.

Can you identify some of the issues and dilemmas that are framed by each person in this scenario?

Under Section 47 of the National Assistance Act 1948 persons who:

(a) are suffering from grave chronic disease or, being aged, infirm or physically incapacitated, are living in insanitary conditions; and
(b) are unable to devote to themselves, and are not receiving from other persons, proper care and attention,

can be compulsorily removed from home. A person can only be detained against his or her will in a place named in the court order. There is no legal aid for representation or requirement that the person be represented or even have legal advice although there is a limited right of appeal.

In terms of anti-oppressive practice it is important to take into account that all parties are given information and made aware of the consequences of compulsory removal and the infringement of people's civil liberties. It is acknowledged that such legislation is draconian and its use should be limited. Compulsion does always carry with it infringement of people's rights. Such principles apply in all legislation which carries compulsory powers.

Societal expectations are that professionals, sometimes in consultation with relatives, will make assessments based on the best interests of the person concerned, as long as these do not conflict with the rights of others. An important principle here is that as far as possible the vulnerable person should be fully involved. Your knowledge of anti-oppressive practice principles will, we hope, have made you instantly aware of the fact that in the above scenario Bill Valentine was not included in the discussion! The power to override the wishes of the vulnerable person or her or his family should not be abused.

> Unless clear statutory authority to the contrary exists, no one is to be detained in hospital or to undergo medical treatment or even to submit himself to a medical examination without his consent. That is as true of a mentally disordered person as of anyone else.
> (McCullough J, in the case of *R* v *Hallstrom* [1986] 2 All ER 314; quoted by Brayne and Martin 1990: 253)

A framework of assessment

From an analysis of some of the above examples we suggest that an ethical framework of assessment needs to include the following points.

1 Assessment should involve those being assessed.
2 Openness and honesty should permeate the process.
3 Assessment should involve the sharing of values and concerns.
4 There should be acknowledgement of the structural context of the process.
5 The process should be about questioning the basis of the reasons for proposed action, and all those involved should consider alternative courses of action.
6 Assessment should incorporate the different perspectives of the people involved.

By way of illustration the following case will be used to demonstrate the above points.

In *Manchester City Council* v *S* (1991) 2 FLR 370, reported in *Family Law*, January 1992, Volume 22, the defendant was the mother of two girls aged 12 and 10 who were made wards of court in February 1989. At the hearing in March 1989 the judge concluded that both children were suffering from psychiatric disorders, which were a consequence of the mother's own problems. Supervised access was ordered at the discretion of the local authority, and a return of the children to the care of the mother if she took appropriate advice and treatment. They were then admitted to a residential home.

At a further hearing in February 1990 the local authority maintained that the problems the children faced were caused by the mother's psychiatric illness. The local authority was granted a full care order but suspended placement pending a further hearing to give the mother the chance to take treatment. Monthly access to the mother was ordered. She attended outpatient sessions with a psychiatrist and a programme to work towards rehabilitation was devised.

By July 1990 the situation looked promising and a recommendation for increased unsupervised access was made – taking place overnight on 28–29 July 1990. But in August 1990 the local authority unilaterally decided that the assessment had broken down and stopped access without any court sanction. Access was then reinstated on a monthly basis at a further hearing in October 1990. In March 1991 the local authority opposed rehabilitation and proposed an alternative long-term placement for the children. However, it later conceded that the welfare of the children demanded that they should return to the care of their mother.

In her judgment, Bracewell J found that staff at the residential home and the social services department had not really been in favour of the assessment with a view to rehabilitation and were quick to attribute the behaviour of the children to increased contact with the mother. Despite the psychiatrist's favourable reports and successful overnight unsupervised access, the local authority appeared to have interpreted matters against the mother, as criticism, when none was justified. Her ladyship therefore found that the assessment had not broken down. She also recommended that a black social worker become involved with the family.

A number of issues concerning the dilemmas of assessment are highlighted by this case.

1 It could be argued that the intervention was justified although the mother did not suffer from any specific mental disorder. The issue was how her personality might or might not affect her ability to parent her children, and if it did adversely affect her ability then whether there was a capacity for change within the time scale of the children's needs.
2 Assessment:
    (a) Was the assessment given a fair chance?
    (b) Did the assessment break down?
3 Partnership:
    (a) Since August 1990, through no fault of her own, the mother had been bereft of assistance; at one period she had access to her children stopped, contrary to the court order, and then reinstated only at monthly intervals; and she had been excluded from any involvement with planning for the children's future.
    (b) There was no clear indication of who was in overall control of managing the case. Court orders and directions did not appear to have been explained by the legal advisors to the local authority or understood by the key worker. There had been a lack of effective communication between staff at the residential home and the social services department.
4 Participation:
    (a) No one had explained to the children the result, significance or consequences of events after February 1990, and in particular the local

authority failed to explain the increased access and then cessation of
access at the time when the assessment was alleged to have failed.

(b) There had been no consideration of the expressed wishes of the children.
(c) The children had been given no effective explanation of the reason for
delays of court hearings.
(d) No planning (Darlow 1992).

The case happened before the implementation of the Children Act 1989.
Lowe (1992) points out that the case should now be better managed as a
result of the legislation, i.e. timetabling, use of orders, partnership, choice
and rights, and greater emphasis on local authority plans for children in
care.

However, it is important to acknowledge the impact that values will have
on the assessment process – if the value base of those involved remains the
same then arguably no amount of change in the legislation will affect the
outcome. For example:

• Was the mother deemed to be an 'unfit' mother by some of the parties
  involved because of her mental health difficulties?
• Were the needs of the children considered in relation to those of the
  mother?
• Was any account taken of the factor of 'race' and how this might have
  affected not only her mental health and that of the children but also how
  other people responded to them?
• Whom did the mother have to advocate for her?
• Whom did the children have to advocate for them?

These questions should have been asked under the old legislation and should
also be asked under the new legislation if the outcome is to be different.

Under the Children Act 1989 there is now no wardship option for the
local authority. If it wants a care order it must apply and make out its case
under Section 31. If the court decides to make a care order it cannot then
add directions to the local authority, but it can make a contact order under
Section 34 and attach conditions to that order (Section 34 (7)). There is also
an obligation on the local authority to seek court sanction for cessation or
restriction of contact. The court must also explore options other than a care
order (Section 1 (3)(g)), including the making of Section 8 orders and/or a
supervision order. Lowe points out that the likelihood is that the court
would have made a care order but with a supervised contact order and with
a further return date to the court. But this, of course, to a greater degree, will
depend on the assessment made by the professionals involved.

The power of assessment in determining change

Within the legislative framework in which we operate a number of assessments are required. For example:

• NHS and Community Care Act 1990, Section 47 deals with assessments
  and care plans for individuals.

- Disabled Persons Act 1986, Sections 3, 4 and 7 make provision for assessment and advocacy, however only Section 4 has been implemented.
- Mental Health Act 1983, admission for assessment Section 2, emergency assessment Section 4 and assessment for treatment Section 3.
- Children Act 1989, assessments need to be undertaken in relation to Part III of the Act.
- Education Act 1993, assessment for statementing of special educational needs.
- Criminal Justice Act 1991, pre-sentence reports are required to 'assist the court in determining the most suitable method of dealing with an offender' (Section 3 (5)(a)).

Sometimes in an assessment other legislation has to be taken into account. For example, following assessment under Section 47 of the Community Care Act 1990 local authorities are obliged to take into account their duties under Section 2 of the Chronically Sick and Disabled Persons Act 1970 and consider other legislation, such as the National Assistance Act 1948, the National Health Service Act 1977 and the Mental Health Act 1983. Assessments relating to children with disabilities can be combined with those under other legislation such as the Education Act 1993, the Disabled Persons Act 1986 and the Chronically Sick and Disabled Persons Act 1970. Once a young person reaches the age of 18 then she or he comes within the Community Care Act 1990.

Given that there are all these opportunities to present people's needs, we are also provided with opportunities to make the detail of people's lives visible. Therefore we need to remind ourselves of the framework of anti-oppressive practice, which we considered in Chapter 7. We make no apologies for reminding you of our discussions in Part I: anti-oppressive assessment involves a process of understanding and comparing the values, attitudes and behaviour of the larger societal system with those of the user's immediate family and community system. This provides the framework of reference for effectual decision making and thus is vital to assessment – it is impossible to assess accurately without that knowledge (Norton 1978).

Final thoughts

The complex nature of assessments cannot be overemphasized. From assessments decisions are made about people's lives. If the assessment process is not underpinned by the principles that inform anti-oppressive practice then the situation of the person being assessed is not truly reflected.

It is important, therefore, that any assessment takes account of the power differentials that exist between both individuals and groups. There must also be some understanding of the links between people's personal experiences of oppression and the structural reality of inequality. As practitioners we must be aware of ourselves in the assessment process and how both we and the service user will inevitably change. That means that we can be in the positions of 'participant' and of 'observer', a process which has been described as 'reflexivity' (Clifford 1994).

Activities

Activity 1

The NHS and Community Care Act 1990 imposes a duty on local authorities to undertake comprehensive and multi-disciplinary assessments which should be needs-led, and involve users and carers in the process. In short the assessment should include: 'assessment of the applicant's circumstances, in the round, and his or her personal needs for support and rehabilitation, including any community service needs, together with any help or support required by carers' (DoH 1991b).

For this activity you need to look at an assessment schedule. You can obtain this from the agency in which you are working or from a local social services office. You can then use the principles below to assess this schedule critically. Alternatively you could talk to someone involved in assessments of older people and carers and try to identify what principles inform his or her practice before comparing them with the five core principles outlined below. If you have been the subject of an assessment you might like to reflect on this experience and consider whether you feel that the core principles informed the process.

At the level of practice in assessing older people and their carers five core principles have been identified:

- begin from the user's and the carer's definitions of the relevant problems or issues;
- be comprehensive, that is, be flexible and adaptable to enable a wide range of factors and information to be collated, as appropriate to each individual person and her or his circumstances;
- provide a coherent framework for understanding and prioritizing the complex information gathered from a range of different sources;
- take account of issues of confidentiality;
- offer a consistent standard of good practice to users and carers while also recognizing that the process of assessment involves the exercising of judgement, whether professional judgement or subjective judgement of users and carers (Hughes 1993).

Activity 2

Read the following account from a woman whose 80-year-old mother is finding it increasingly difficult to carry on in the role of carer. Her specific practical needs are for help getting into and out of bed and with washing and dressing.

I get the district nurse to come in. Of course she has to come in to do the catheter but she's not the person to help give me a wash down below and help me get into the chair you know – it has to be another person. Now the other person that comes in to get me into the chair is not allowed to wash me. I've never heard anything like it in my life. We had a meeting here on Thursday of the social services person, the home help person, the physiotherapist and my district nurse, and each one had a different job and one can't go over and do the other person's job. And when she said that the person who's coming to help me, she's coming Monday to Friday – she can dress me, she can get me out of bed but she's not allowed to wash me. And I said well who's allowed to wash me then? . . . So if ever you're out and you smell something, it will be a smelly paraplegic. Oh dear, oh dear, these rules and regulations.

(Zarb 1991)

What does this tell you about:

- the assessment;
- the coordination of resources;
- needs-led/resource-led dilemmas within the assessment process;
- multi-disciplinary working?

During the course of our life we are all assessed for different services. Think about the last time you were asked a series of questions.

- Did you feel that they were relevant?
- Did you feel that your privacy was invaded?
- Did you have the opportunity to ask questions about the service?
- Were you asked why you felt that you needed the particular service?
- Did you understand the questions asked?

10   PLANNING

It sounded like an excellent plan, no doubt, and very neatly and simply arranged; the only difficulty was, that she had not the smallest idea how to set about it . . .
(Lewis Carroll, Alice's Adventures in Wonderland)

Two people in a day centre:

'I've been assessed but I don't know what happens next.'

'Oh, you have to wait a bit and then everyone has a meeting to see what they can do. They never say you can have what you need though.'

'Oh I know that! Do you remember Mabel. She wanted someone to wash her and she had all kinds of people in the meeting you know – the health visitor, the social worker and goodness knows who else – but none of them could do what she needed.'

Two young people in a children's home:

'My social worker said I've been assessed but I've just got to wait now.'

'After I was assessed they said they couldn't find a place in the country to suit me, so now they're assessing me again.'

'So what's the point of assessing you again if you've already been assessed.'

'So they can find somewhere that's OK, I guess.'

Medical practitioner and assistant director of social services:

'I'm sick and tired of being told that I can't place my patients in my nursing home. I just don't know what this community care stuff is all about.'

'I don't know how you can say you don't know about it. We've put ourselves out to set up seminars, provide you with briefing sessions, everyone has had personal letters, newsletters. If I remember rightly you were even on one of the working parties!'

The language of social care practice is now more focused on planning. We talk about *care plans* and *planning meetings* in relation to young people and vulnerable adults. Local authorities produce service and development plans, care planning documents, community care plans and so on – all as a result of the legislation, and in recognition of the importance of planning. What does all this mean? What does it mean to service users? What does it mean to workers? What does it mean to those who have to produce policy and practice strategies?

We will consider these questions by first looking at planning in legislation and the use of assessments to assist in the planning process. In an exploration of routes to and through clienthood and the use of written agreements we will consider the implications for service users and workers. Finally, we will discuss conflicts that can arise between needs and services.

Planning in the legislation

One of the better known pieces of recent legislation is the National Health Service and Community Care Act 1990, which requires local authorities to prepare and publish plans for the provision of community care services (Section 46). Health departments and social services departments have had to establish joint care planning teams to advise on the development of strategic plans. The plans are intended to meet the needs of such groups as 'dependent elderly people, those with disabilities whether of a learning, physical or sensory nature and those affected by HIV/AIDS or women suffering domestic violence' (DoH 1990). The intention of this section is that authorities will respond to the identified needs of the communities they serve rather than plan the services that they think people should want: this links in with the social justice model approach to service provision. The plan should respond to expressed needs even when only a few people are demanding a particular service.

In addition to this the Act provides for each individual to have her or his needs assessed (Section 47) and the guidance states that 'all users in receipt of a continuous service should have a care plan' (DoH 1991b: para. 4.1). There is an obligation to assess needs, but meeting them is discretionary. However, discretion also gives a degree of power, so that logically assessment should lead to a plan.

Other legislation and its associated guidance also indicates the importance of planning (e.g. the Children Act 1989, the Criminal Justice Act 1991).

Using the assessments for planning

In order to ensure that our assessments are based on need we must know what value framework informs our definition of need. This definition can be

framed either in the context of individual pathology or within a social justice model. If we assess using an individual pathology model then it will
only fit the specific situation and we are more likely to try to fit needs to
available services rather than tailor services to needs. The social justice model,
however, recognizes inequalities within society and attempts to provide services which will challenge them. So how we assess and the plans we make are
determined by our understanding of need. In looking back at assessments,
therefore, it is important that we take account of the social inequalities that
exist and that we should 'beware of imposing middle-class, sexist, heterosexist,
disabilist, ageist or other stereotypical norms upon our assessments' (Clifford
1994: 226).

Brayne and Martin (1990) liken planning to a map which we need to
follow in order to complete a journey. They point out that if we are asked
for directions we can't respond with a vague 'It's five miles away, sort of
north from here', but must give exact details of landmarks, road names and
numbers, traffic lights, roundabouts and so on. Equally, it is no use saying
that 'we hope that we can get there by going sort of north'; we need to know
exactly where we are going and how much fuel we have. This requires a
map. 'There' can be anything from needing a nursery place for an individual
child to providing a housing scheme for black elders. Having completed the
assessment, we need to consider the issues that are raised and work out an
appropriate map to follow.

Routes to and through clienthood

Perhaps the map we are drawing is the next stage of a journey that was
started long before any interaction with workers in an agency. Payne (1993:
169) argues that when a client seeks assistance from a social care agency he
or she may well have already followed a 'circuitous pathway'. This pathway
is what Malcolm Payne calls the *route to clienthood*, which, he argues, is a
process that continues as a route *through* clienthood while that person has
contact with an agency.

It is therefore a valuable part of any early assessment to consider someone's route to clienthood, as this defines the nature of the work which may
be undertaken with that person, and thus the planning. What she or he
wants will actually be defined by the route. In practice, workers will be able
to be more effective in their interactions if they concern themselves about
the route to the agency. The effectiveness of the service will also be affected
by the different kinds of clienthood that people experience when receiving
services and how they understand the route onward.

One of the reasons why such an understanding is necessary is the frag-
mentation of services and the creation of the contract–provider split that has
arisen from the National Health Service and Community Care Act 1990.
Instead of an older person receiving social work, home help, mobile meals
and day care all from the social services department, he or she may well
receive them from various agencies in the statutory and voluntary or private
sectors.

Both workers and users of the services will need to come to terms with the relationships between these services and the rationales within which they operate. Payne points out, for example, that a client may find it difficult to accept a service from a voluntary agency, seeing it as 'charity', and prefer to be treated as a customer by buying in a commercial service. Others may feel they have a right to a service and resent the privatization of what was formerly a statutory service. Furthermore, when a client needs to move on from these services into residential care there may be problems in delivering an accustomed service (e.g. a trusted GP or a continuing occupational therapy service) into a private residential facility. This is because public services are not allowed or are actively discouraged by the home's managers.

The status of 'client' can also be complex and uncertain depending on how people are defined and by whom – and this will also affect planning. Coming back briefly to consideration of language, we can see that changes in legislation and the principles underlying it can affect the terminology we use. As we noted in Chapter 6, social workers have traditionally referred to people to whom they offer services as 'clients', but the same people may also be patients to health service practitioners – with whom social workers may be in a close working relationship. 'Patient' has been seen to imply a less autonomous status.

In other agencies, especially in the voluntary sector, they may be called 'users', with implications that they have more autonomy and choice. However, there are also problems with this word, which has been criticized because it has associations with drug users. It has been seen as a consumerist term with Citizen's Charter connotations which assumes a false sense of equality (see Chapter 6). Finally, it can be criticized in relation to compulsory intervention, where people are not in receipt of services by choice but are called users (e.g. a young person in residential care on an Emergency Protection Order or a person detained under mental health legislation).

Use of the word 'customer' or 'consumer' is preferred by other agencies to emphasize the purchasing-of-service relationship, giving more control of services offered and the right to stop buying that service. It has been suggested that use of the word 'consumer' is preferable to use of 'user' because 'with its market-place connotations [it] seems a more accurate representation of the "active citizen" model favoured by the present government' (Phillips *et al.* 1994: 129).

The notion of status is further complicated by the fact that some clients may, for example, be considered as colleagues. With the principles of participation and partnership underpinning both legislation and anti-oppressive practice, gone is the clear-cut distinction between client and colleague. At one time 'clients were helped and colleagues were co-operators in helping' (Payne 1993: 172). Now clients may invariably be seen as participants and colleagues in the process. Even then, though, it is not straightforward.

Payne gives as an example foster carers, who may be regarded as colleagues but are often offered support in similar ways to clients – such support, however, furthers the work of the agency, rather than making the carer the object of its help. Another example is that of a parent of an adult with learning difficulties, who may be treated as a colleague in helping the client, be a part of the family which is seen as the client or be a client in her or his own right in trying to cope with the stress of caring. Through a sophisticated understanding of clienthood, combining 'process' and 'status', we come to see the term as signifying a changing state with changing roles, 'involving a complex interaction with the agency and other players in the community and related agencies' (Payne 1993: 176).

There is a need for a clear understanding of the roles of the players at any stage, particularly in terms of planning the action. We will now think about how to involve people in the planning process. One way of involving clients in planning the service that they require to meet their needs is through the use of written agreements.

The use of written agreements

A written agreement, if used within a relationship that is based on partnership, will be a useful practice tool. The use of such an agreement is based on an enabling rather than a directive approach, which empowers those we work with, because it promotes user involvement and control (Croft and Beresford 1993). Written and negotiated agreements between people and practitioners should promote an exchange of views, 'minimise misunderstanding and counter some of the negative effects of being a recipient or user of social services' (Braye and Preston-Shoot 1993: 38).

The use of written agreements has become more accepted as a way of working as a result of some more recent legislation. Although there is nothing in legislation about the use of written agreements, guidance and regulations have clear expectations that they will be made and recommend what should be included in such agreements. Young people, for example, should now have a care plan and this should be drawn up in writing in the form of an agreement. In its widest sense it takes the form of a contract which can involve a number of people, e.g. the young person, those with parental responsibility, relevant carers and other agencies.

Supervision of Probation Orders should also work to an individual *supervision plan*, which should 'wherever possible be *agreed* with the offender and *signed* by both the offender and supervising officer' (Department of Health and the Welsh Office 1992: 38). The offender is then given a copy of the plan. Home Office guidance in this respect states very clearly what the plans should contain and the importance of regular reviewing of the plan, and if, after the review the plan is revised, then, 'as initially, further copies of the plan should be given to the offender' (Department of Health and the Welsh Office 1992: 38).

Similarly, guidance for community care plans states that they should be set out in 'concise written form' and be accessible to the user, such as in braille or translated into the user's own language. A copy should be given to the user but it should also, subject to the constraints of confidentiality, be shared with other contributors to the plan' (DoH 1991b: 67). The accessibility of written agreements is essential if they are to be effective. This is recognized in the community care guidance and it is also a point made by Ryan (1994: 157):

Families welcome the use of written agreements because the openness that they require is preferable to their having to rely on the goodwill of professionals or their relationship with the social worker. If necessary, agreements could and should be recorded in ways other than, or in addition to, writing. For example, by using a videotape, audio cassette, braille or computer disc.

Planning in action

George Workard is an experienced white social worker who is trying to get to grips with the new child care planning document the department has just issued: it is 30 pages long and to him just seems to be full of boxes and lots of space to fill in! George is a respected social worker, but his colleagues will joke with him about the mound of files that overflow on his desk. The constant cry from George from behind the mountain of papers is 'I really must get my write-ups done!'

Two weeks ago he visited the Crossroads family following an initial referral by Mrs Crossroads, who is a white mother concerned about her ten-year-old son, Peter, who is black and subjected to racial abuse both in and outside school. Outside school the abuse comes from one particular family. The children of this family attend the same school as Peter. Mr and Mrs Crossroads have recently separated. Peter is now starting to find reasons for not going to school.

That morning George's team manager mentions to George that he has supervision the next morning. This reminds him that he must complete the planning document and agreement within 30 days of receiving the initial referral. He decides to call in on his way back from another visit that morning. Armed with his document he is a bit put out when Mrs Crossroads informs him that she is on the way to the nursery to collect her youngest child.

Comment: Although there is pressure of time, George should be aware that respect for the people involved demands that proper appointments are made and that time is allocated to successful completion of the task. Furthermore, it is essential that everyone is consulted and involved in making the plan and drawing up the agreement if the plan is to have any chance of success. The Children Act 1989 requires that in work with children in need and their families the responsible authority should reach agreement on the plan with the parents or those with parental responsibility and the child where appropriate (Regulations 3 and 4).

Having made an appointment, George starts to talk about the problem as seen by the family. Peter becomes restless and a little agitated and starts to wander about. He says to George, 'Have you come to talk to me about my dad?' Eventually he asks his mother whether he can go to his room. She says 'Yes'. George doesn't intervene, as the document weighs heavily on his lap.

Comment: For a parent and child to give informed consent there must be a common understanding of the problem(s), which involves an open and full discussion with everyone concerned. The situation involves not just filling in a form but ascertaining the wishes, feelings and needs of all those involved, especially Peter. His life experiences which include racism must inform the plan.

George suggests that perhaps it would be a good idea for him to talk to Peter's teacher. Peter's Mum welcomes this as she thinks it would be helpful if the school knows how her son is feeling and perhaps helps in some way. At this point Peter returns to the room and is obviously angry. He shouts at George that he doesn't want the school to know anything about his life, it's none of their business.

Comment: George is aware that the legislation talks about working in partnership with other agencies and therefore feels he should involve the school. However, the legislation also stresses that young people should be fully consulted and their wishes and feelings taken into account. Peter's feelings must be respected. To inform the school of social work involvement with Peter would clearly be difficult for him given his feelings. But it is important that the school is aware of the racism which Peter is encountering there and has the opportunity to address it. A way forward, then, could be for George to talk generally with the headteacher about the issue of racism within the school and how this could be addressed.

George recognizes from Peter's response that he has feelings about the situation but – as a white worker – is unsure about how to proceed. He talks to Peter and his mother about various options, which include consultation with another black worker, involvement of Peter in a support group and help for Mrs Crossroads, who is anxious to help her son. George is also mindful of the difficulties he might face in trying to get these services. It then dawns on him that a written agreement would be useful to provide him with a bargaining tool to attempt to secure resources.

Comment: The philosophy behind the whole child care planning document is to collect statistical information about needs in order to be able to provide appropriate services. It also enables a strategic child care policy to be developed which is sensitive to the community served by the authority. Even if George is unable to provide the services identified in the plan immediately he does have a written document which provides the necessary evidence to secure future resources.

Managing the conflict between needs and services

The legislation embodies within it a vision of the needs of individuals which will enable them to achieve their full potential. The concept of need is informed by a particular value base, which can be clearly seen in relation to the NHS and Community Care Act 1990: services are provided on the basis of need rather than the fact that as an older or vulnerable person you have the right to a service.

Need is based on an individual pathology model rather than a social justice model. There is a tension, therefore, if you are working from an empowerment perspective and a social justice model, with the legislation, which operates on an individual 'medical model of welfare' (Braye and Preston-Shoot 1992a). If you are working with an individual, but informed by a social justice perspective, your assessment of need and the consequent planning of services to meet that need should be focused on extending and improving the range and quality of the existing service provision, rather than on overcoming the deficits of individuals and their families. Your individual work should contribute to the process of change. It is not about *taking services off the shelf* but about taking account of the need that is identified and providing the services to meet that need.

Sapey and Hewitt (1991) point out that since 'need' is not clearly defined, and social care practitioners are left to assess the needs of individuals, there is scope to make these assessments as wide as one's imagination will allow. A proper assessment can thus ensure that people are entitled to services that are not necessarily incorporated into agency definitions or procedures. Sapey and Hewitt state, for example, that it is important to interpret the language of legislation in a way that will ensure that disabled people are not further disabled by the concept of need. The purpose of needs-led assessment, therefore, must be understood by the worker. If it is not, then only an individual service is provided, whereas the information gathered should be collated to promote a service which meets all needs.

'Care planning is just about ticking boxes. There are no resources to meet the needs, so what is the point of doing it?' This was the comment of one worker in a hospital social work team who feels pressurized by time and lack of resources. She argues that she is assessing what people need in terms of physical resources rather than perhaps helping them to understand what their lives will be like once they leave hospital. Social workers in such situations feel disempowered because they consider that what they are doing is an administrative task, i.e. organizing resources rather than using their skills as practitioners. They feel powerless because all they can see are finite resources, complex needs and no solutions.

It could be said that the job of professionals is to ration the resources to meet needs identified through the legislation. A similar argument has been put forward in discussions about meeting the needs of disabled people (Sapey and Hewitt 1991). Local authorities have legislative powers and duties to deliver the services that Parliament considers will reduce disabling environments. However, many workers feel that they are agents of social control and merely police disability. Until workers move from seeing disability as an individual problem to seeing it as a collective one, and discard medical models, they will continue to collude with procedures which limit people's access to resources they control. Social care practitioners in such situations see themselves as gatekeepers. They decide who does or does not deserve a service, rather than empowering people to determine their own needs. Social care practice, however, 'operates at the interface of legislation, between implementers of that legislation, attitudes of society and disabled people' (Sapey and Hewitt 1991: 41).

Local authorities can only operate within a legislative framework. Expenditure and income has to be within the powers and duties laid down in that legislation. But there can be broad interpretations. For example, the National Assistance Act 1948 permits expenditure on residential and day care facilities, but there is also a general duty towards the 'welfare' of service users. The notion of welfare changes, however, as societal attitudes and political thinking changes. So, it has been suggested, the role of local authorities can be quite dramatically affected; for instance, the move away from institutional care of people with learning difficulties (Sapey and Hewitt 1991).

It is not impossible to overcome financial constraints in order to improve quality. In one review of service and development plans that we read the following points were made.

It was generally recognised that there are not endless funds available to meet all the needs identified. Equally, it was felt that financial constraints should not be viewed as a negative factor or a reason for not trying to get things done. Indeed, it was thought that the overall quality of services could be improved by implementing many of the recommended developments and in particular:

- encouraging different agencies to work together and pool resources and expertise;
- regular reviews of services to see whether they could be provided more efficiently;
- better overall coordination in order to minimise duplication of effort and expenditure;
- recognising the needs of the whole communities and not just 'pockets'.
(Rochdale Metropolitan Borough Council 1993)

Obviously it is important not to accept too readily the argument put forward by conservative policies that we should 'spend less, and more wisely'. But the above points do provide a guide to the direction in which service planners and workers should be heading. A commitment to a shared understanding of the need to plan appropriate, flexible services jointly is required if change is to be effective.

Final thoughts

The achievement of a needs-led approach to the planning and delivery of services is dependent on practitioners undertaking comprehensive and multi-disciplinary assessments of individuals who require a service. The Children Act 1989 and the National Health Service and Community Care Act 1990 have set into action work within health and social welfare departments that is focused upon meeting the needs of the communities in which they are based. The emphasis on *working together* has led to the development of partnership arrangements within local authorities. This is a positive and essential move for effective planning.

We would argue that if the 'needs' of the community are to be met then it is important to review and evaluate existing service provision as well as to undertake research in order to ascertain existing need. By profiling the community, which can be done through the analysis of information provided by census details, service planners are provided with a picture of the levels and nature of deprivation faced by local communities. From this overview an understanding is drawn of various communities' experiences of oppression, and appropriate plans can be made regarding the allocation of resources and the development and delivery of services.

Research into the needs of communities in order to plan effectively is not, it appears, always undertaken by service providers. For example, it is only in recent times that the importance of planning for children has been promoted. An overview of research studies published by the DoH in 1991 stated that

> Research findings indicate that considerable progress has been made in establishing the importance of planning for children and some success achieved in putting it into practice, although disturbing instances of lack of plans are also mentioned in a number of the SSI and other reports.
>
> (DoH 1991a: 64)

Evidence from research supports the view that planning, if it is to be effective and of good quality, should incorporate the active involvement of users. It is also essential to set realistic aims and objectives – the legislation provides the impetus for action in this direction.

Activity

The Children Act 1989 and the NHS and Community Care Act 1990 both identify the importance of a negotiated and planned service provision. Refer back to the scenario with George and Peter that we outlined earlier. George manages to visit on two further occasions and gathers more information to make an assessment, in partnership with Peter and his mother. He then draws up a plan and written agreement. Put yourself in George's position and draw up an appropriate plan and agreement.

Commentary
The Children Act 1989 states very clearly that each child and/or family should have a clear plan. The guidance and the regulations give a comprehensive list of what should be considered in developing the plan.

Plans should be written in clear, easily understood language. The agreement then follows on from the plan and will list the specific aims and objectives which will be acted upon, and by whom. Everyone involved in the agreement should receive a copy of it.

If they are drawn up as a part of a true partnership then written agreements can be empowering. If a plan is not followed, the resources have not been provided as agreed or a decision is made which is contrary to the agreement, then the user can complain through the local authority complaints procedure. If the user feels that the agreement is not fair, or that he or she has not been fully involved in the process, then he or she should be able to appeal against the contents of the agreement through the complaints procedure. In the case of Peter, for instance, if the agreement is made without his involvement, then he has a genuine complaint.

11 WORKING WITH OR

FOR USERS

They said he couldn't be gay
They said he couldn't love
They said he couldn't care
They said he couldn't have feelings
They said he couldn't show emotions
They said he couldn't until he was eighteen.
They said he had to wait –
And be something he's not.
Everybody who decided, were straight
So how could they know?
You cannot put a limit on feelings,
Obviously that's what they've done.
What happens to the opinion
Of the men who are actually gay?
Where was their involvement
In the decisions that were made?
The people who it affects
Should have played a large part in the say.

(Chrissie Elms Bennett 1994)

The principles of participation underpin much current legislation and thinking in health and social care practice. In this chapter we will explore how
we can work with users in ways which are not patronizing or tokenistic. It
has been suggested that the 'rhetoric of participation reflects only a capacity
to refuse rather than change what is offered' (Payne 1993: 172) and it has
proved difficult to put true participation into practice (Croft and Beresford
1992). The question 'is user involvement a good thing?' is no longer up for
debate. It is firmly on the agenda. It is demanded by user organizations and
required by legislation (Croft and Beresford 1992). There is no reason to
assume that legislation such as the Community Care Act (1990) can bring

about significant change. However, the White Paper *Caring for People* (DoH 1989) did envisage a change in the nature of service provision, including user participation, involvement in inspections and quality assurance, consultation in community care planning and complaints procedures, which we will discuss in more detail in the course of the chapter.

Values

Croft and Beresford (1993) have suggested that there are eight key elements which contribute to making user involvement for organizations and services a reality.

1 *Resources.* Involving people requires resources (both material and human) and this has to be recognized by those seeking to promote genuine participation.
2 *Information.* Information is power and needs to be shared. To be effective information should:

- be of immediate relevance, clear, attractive and brief;
- be appropriate to people's abilities, experience, knowledge, language and culture;
- take into account particular needs of members of minority ethnic communities, people with limited ability, people with sensory disabilities, people with limited literacy skills;
- link verbal and written information;
- be available from clear contact points;
- offer the chance to get to know the information given, to develop trust and confidence.

3 *Training.* Participation will be tokenistic if there is no acknowledgement that people have skills but these need to be developed through training. Professionals have had access to specialized training in order to carry out their tasks. In order to empower people to be able to participate on an equal footing they must also have access to training. This does not mean that participation should be conditional on training, but there needs to be a recognition that we all have training needs. The best training is where everyone is involved together and users contribute to the training process.
4 *Research and evaluation.* Obviously it would be contrary to the whole notion of participation not to involve users in any research undertaken or evaluation of services and projects.
5 *Equal access and opportunities.* People cannot say something about services unless they have access to them.
6 *Forums and structures for involvement.* It is important to have participatory structures and forums where people can feel comfortable about airing their views.
7 *Language.* Language is not neutral and we should check out that we all have a common understanding of what is being said.

8 *Advocacy*. There are many forms of advocacy, which ensure that people who are in receipt of services have a voice that is respected and valued. This ensures that the views of users are listened to and acknowledged.

These guiding principles can be used to help us, through the framework of the law, to work positively with users. We wrote in Chapter 3 about the importance of knowing our own value base and understanding that of the law. Such principles are informed by an empowerment perspective and user involvement can only be effective if our value base can accept and acknowledge those principles.

Values in action

Stockport Social Services Division Children's Services Plan commences with a statement of values and principles of the division's services to children and young people and their families. Along with all social services departments Stockport is required to construct such plans (DoH 1992a). The statement is based on principles underpinning the legislation and consists of a series of points under three headings.

Under the heading *'Children and young people'* there are ten points, of which the following is an example: 'Services and young people are disadvantaged in a society where power is predominantly experienced by adults and males. Services should recognise this and seek to empower children and young people more' (1.4). There are eight points under the heading *'Parents and families'*. For example: 'Parenting is stressful, and this stress is exacerbated by a range of social and environmental pressures. Poverty and poor housing are particularly significant factors that create stress that has an adverse effect on the care of children and young people' (2.2). Finally, there are twelve points under the heading *'Social services division'*. For example: 'Services for children and their families should be visible, accessible and understandable in practical terms to all the cultures and communities they serve and be responsive to their needs' (3.9).

At the end of this comprehensive statement the reader has a clear understanding of the value base informing the authority's practice. Furthermore, the statement is followed by an anti-oppressive practice statement and commitments which identify the framework within which work with children and families is conducted.

Such statements must be an integral part of any service plans – by both statutory and voluntary agencies – for there to be total commitment to user involvement in the planning and provision of services. From each statement effective action should be developed.

Values and the contract culture

Clear position statements, as outlined above, enable service providers to have some control over how they engage with others. Because such statements need to be publicized users should have a clear understanding of what their relationship will be to the service provider. Service provision is now within the market place – even though we may not agree with the ideology of the mixed market economy and may, like Walby (1993: 356), feel that there are 'clear dangers in the uncritical pursuit of the contract culture'. We have to acknowledge the fact that we have to live with it and work within it.

It has been suggested that the mixed economy of care will increase user choice. Evidence from research suggests that it is usually the voluntary organizations that, having already demonstrated an ability to provide services, are encouraged to develop services to meet identified need (Lart and Taylor 1993). This does result in a service preferred by users but does not increase user choice. Purchasing authorities must therefore seek to attract a variety of providers into the market place and use resources to this end if real choices are to be available to users. Sometimes practitioners may find some of the choices of service users controversial. They may then choose not to actively put in the appropriate service, preferring to use what they have and 'add on'.

Josephine's story highlights this very point. Josephine was a young lesbian woman who particularly wanted to be fostered with a lesbian couple and also wanted counselling from a lesbian worker. The worker was aware of the existence of a specialized service for young gays and lesbians but the authority would not support any official contact with this agency. It preferred to use existing service provision and to bring in a counsellor who was known to have an interest in this area. Although Josephine had a service her voice was not listened to and she had no real choice.

Our role, then, is to seek out other services and stimulate provision which is flexible to meet users' needs. But this is no easy task. If we look at the position of voluntary organizations they are themselves ambiguous about entering into agreements with local authorities if their ideals are then compromised by the purchaser. For example, an agency providing counselling for young gays and lesbians had to provide a child protection policy before it could obtain local authority funding, which contradicted its own confidentiality policy. If we are committed to the tenets of user involvement, though, we must strive to provide flexible service provision in order to maximize choice.

Empowerment: access to files

One of the steps towards empowerment of users is the sharing of information. A concrete way of sharing information is through access to one's records. Sharing of records equalizes the relationship between the users and the provider of a service and enhances participation. The Access to Personal Files Act 1987 gave the right to service users to see their personal files. It also provided the impetus for work within social welfare agencies to be a 'more open activity' (Payne 1989: 114).

The practice of sharing decisions with users and opening up records presents a number of ethical issues demonstrating the difficulties that workers face when they attempt to work within a participatory framework. The access to records debate highlights the importance of working in partnership with users. Record keeping should, of necessity, involve users' views if records are to be used to guide and inform practice decisions. However, workers can find it difficult to share information honestly with users when the relationship is an unequal one, particularly where information is gathered for the purpose of evidence (e.g. child abuse, elder abuse).

Despite these problems we would argue that if involvement with users is to be successful then the power relationships that exist between users and service providers have to be minimized. One way of attempting to do this is by sharing recorded information. Knowledge of recorded information is the means by which users can verify what is written about them and their situation and correct inaccurate information. It gives back control to users and so aids the process of recovery. Finally, but importantly, sharing information in an open and honest way demonstrates respect.

Issues of accountability to the user and to the agency are also addressed by access to files policies. Assessments and plans are subject to critical evaluation, which is an important aspect of the development of an ethical practice. 'Greater openness and sharing in decision making reflects a greater preparedness to be flexible about the acceptable norms in social work interactions' (Payne 1989: 132). The legislation governing access to records exists and it needs to be actively used to ensure that work with users is based on true partnership and accountability. The eight points for user involvement apply equally to access to records as to any other area of work with users.

Partnership

Involving young people in the decision making processes

This section focuses specifically on work with young people although much of what is written can be transferred to other user groups. The reason for focusing on young people is that they are a powerless group in relation to adults and have consistently been denied full rights to participation by those with power. Hodgson (1990) has suggested that participation involves *information, consultation* and *choice*. A key message in the Children Act 1989 is that young people should be involved in the decisions that are made about their lives. Many workers will say, of course, that they involve young people in decisions. They talk to them about what is happening, they give them the relevant information, they invite them to case conferences, reviews and planning meetings. But is this real participation or is it tokenism?

Let us consider the three areas of information, consultation and choice in a little more detail.

Information

As we have said, information is power. Often young people do not have the information they need. It takes time to ensure that young people do know what is happening and often barriers are created effectively to deny them information. Use of language is an example of this. Feedback from young people who attended a conference organized by the Children's Rights Development Unit included the comment that 'Adults should be very careful about not using jargon and complicated language' (Children's Rights Development Unit 1992: 18). Similar comments were recorded in a survey of young people who attended their case conferences: 'They all used big words like "hypothesis" (I asked Mum after we came out)'; 'You'd need to be as old as my Mum to understand' (Mittler 1992).

A significant piece of research which reflects the voices of young people is the Dolphin Project, which brings together the views of 45 young people who had extensive careers in the care system. The project took place in the summer of 1992. Talking about their participation at reviews, young people identified that they felt intimidated by large meetings. On occasions they would have preferred not to have certain people there, but felt unable to say so. As one person in the project pointed out, this sums up the lack of participation. What makes it worse is that all these people invariably have a set of reports which tells them all about the life of a young person without her or his permission.

Further pointers to good practice are highlighted by Barford and Wattam's research:

> One way to incorporate children further in the process is to disseminate information more effectively, and establish recognisable channels of communication for children. One respondent said she did not mind that she was not allowed to attend the case conference, but she would have liked a copy of the minutes for example.
>
> (Barford and Wattam 1991: 101)

Consultation

At the conference on young people's rights mentioned earlier, those attending were encouraged to be involved in the whole process. These are some of their comments after the event:

> Some of the adults only listened out of politeness and would move on to another subject as soon as you finished talking.

> The adults may have found it interesting to hear our views but we didn't really get anything out of it.

> In our group they jumped from one extreme to another – saying 'let's have a young person's opinion' and we, at the time, would not necessarily have an opinion and when we did have something to say we were ignored.
>
> (CRDU 1992: 18)

If young people feel like this in a conference with adults who are committed to consulting with young people and promoting their rights then what chance do young people have in a more hostile environment? This example clearly illustrates how powerful institutional oppression can be – in this instance the young people are experiencing 'adultism', which 'has the same power dimension as sexism and racism' (Barford and Wattam 1991: 99). The law provides the opportunities for involvement but adults have to be prepared to give up power. User involvement, then, needs very careful planning and for young people must not be done within an adult frame of reference.

Collective action can be a way of assisting users to be heard. But this is only possible if the law is not manipulated by those with the power. In February 1992 Leeds Social Services Department decided to close Gledhow Grange residential home for young people. It was clear that the department had failed to consider the welfare of the young people before making any decision. The young people protested and the outcome of their protest was the creation of a set of consultation procedures. However, as the solicitor representing the children explained,

> the Act clearly states that you consult first and then make a decision based on that consultation. Leeds SSD made a decision and then consulted. It is important that children's wishes are seen to be taken seriously.
>
> (*Community Care*, 24 September 1992)

Whatever situation we are in, whether we are seeing young people in the casualty department of a hospital, talking to them in the classroom, going with them to court, fostering them or in one of the many other situations where we find ourselves working with children and young people, we must always bear in mind that consultation involves listening and taking their views seriously. If the voices of young people are to become established in practice then attitudes of professionals must dramatically change. Otherwise the commitment of the Act to user involvement will never materialize.

Choice

Headlines about young people 'divorcing' their parents accompanied the first attempts of young people to use the Children Act 1989 to their own advantage and to exercise choice within the legal framework. It is sad to see the lives of young people torn apart by adults in their lives, whether in public or private law proceedings. Those who resort to the law are exercising their right to make their own choices. However, for a young person to do this indicates her or his frustration at the lack of opportunity they have to make choices in other arenas. Hodgson (1990) reminds us that 'exercising choice is crucial to the development of children's sense of responsibility', yet it seems that often workers and carers are not prepared to allow young people to make choices and risk making mistakes. Allowing young people choices inevitably means that there has to be recognition of acceptable risk.

Involving parents in the decision making processes

Partnership with parents and child protection procedures do not sit easily together. How can parents be involved and exercise choice in such situations? Research undertaken by Marsh and Fisher (1992) resulted in the development of a set of partnership principles which could be used as a framework for practice:

- Any investigation of problems must be with the explicit consent of the potential user and client, or kept to the minimum necessary by law to assess risks.
- User agreement or a clear statutory mandate is the only basis for partnership based intervention.
- Intervention must be based on the views of all the relevant family members and carers.
- Services must be based on negotiated agreements rather than assumptions and/or prejudices concerning the behaviour and wishes of users.
- Users must have the greatest possible degree of choice in the services they are offered.

Townsend (1992) reminds us of the difficulties that can occur in promoting partnership within the case conference arena. For example, there is the insidious personal identification of staff involved in protecting the child, in front of parents who have done the opposite. Perhaps more obviously, there are the police who have problems discussing potential criminal evidence with an alleged abuser. Doctors and health visitors are likely to give a very sparse account of their perception of the issues. Then there may be the parent who makes a racist, sexist, disabilist, homophobic or other discriminatory remark, who gets very angry and upset at the whole proceedings. Two parents may have a personal slanging match as they blame each other for the situation. And then, of course, there are always grandparents and lawyers to defend various positions.

Townsend (1992: 25) suspects that 'when the Children Act became law, trailing clouds of goodwill and love all round, not to mention hundreds of regulations and bits of advice', the reality of such situations was not considered. Nevertheless, we are rightly required to involve parents in the process – from giving them initial information, right through any investigation to involvement in the conference and any subsequent plans. It is not an easy process and it is worth considering the following questions:

- What does the law require of us?
- What is the primary purpose of any case conference?
- How significant are conferences within the total process?
- What do we mean by the term 'parent'?
- What are the advantages of increased parental participation for children (Fallon 1992: 25)?

Despite Townsend's misgivings, Bell's research, which looked at the involvement of parents in initial child protection conferences, found that the advantages of parental involvement fell broadly into four bands.

- Parental involvement was seen to improve the quality of the information shared. They corrected wrong information, added information and clarified facts. The professionals' contribution was thought to be more carefully worded, objective and relevant, and backed up by evidence.
- Chairing skills were said to be sharper, with the chair person maintaining a focus on the primary purpose of the conference.

- Professionals thought that involvement meant that parents were less likely to scapegoat a particular agency because they would perceive the decision as shared.
- Assessment and treatment plans were perceived as more realistic because of the dialogue with parents during the conference. Forty-five per cent of the sample considered that the net effect of these factors was to enhance the consideration of risk (Bell 1993: 2).

Final thoughts

Although participation is firmly on the agenda, research indicates that often service users feel unable to participate either in the decision making processes which concern their lives or in influencing service provision. While the concept of user involvement might be on our agenda as workers, service providers and carers, it is important that we work at the pace of users. True user involvement must be user-led.

For users to be fully involved practitioners have to recognize and acknowledge the power differences that exist and seek to minimize those differences. Minimizing differences requires us to develop strategies that are based on support from managers and colleagues and understanding from service users (Harding 1993). For strategies to be successful there needs to be recognition of the *opposing* and *supporting* factors which impinge on the process of involving users. For example, one of the *opposing forces* is the unequal power relationships and differing value perspectives that exist between professionals and their colleagues and professionals and service users. *Supporting forces* include the commitment to user involvement, and the relinquishing of power.

It *is* possible to involve users in decision making processes. As Harding (1993), writing about how services can become more user-centred, points out: 'Organisations must also take a closer look at the ways they work which exclude people: the daunting meetings, the incomprehensible language, the pre-ordained objectives and timetable.'

Activity

Angelica is 12 years old. Her mother is Irish and her father is Jamaican. She is a very pretty girl who could 'pass as white'. She has been in a children's home since she was 18 months old when her mother went to Ireland temporarily; her father had previously deserted the family. On her return to England her mother visited Angelica sporadically but was not sufficiently settled to provide a home for her. The plan is that Angelica will eventually be reunited with her mother.

The staff in the children's home where she was placed are mainly white. This pretty child with long plaits is well liked by the staff as she presents no behavioural problems. At the last review it was decided that Angelica should be placed in a foster home, and discussions about the kind of placement are taking place. First, the residential social worker and Angelica discuss the kind of home she would like. Secondly, the field worker and Angelica have a discussion, and then all three together. The field worker raises the subject of a black family, but Angelica and the residential social worker do not feel that this is a good idea: a family, yes; a black one, no.

The task is for you as the person involved in working with Angelica to prepare her for the next review. Whether you are the residential social worker or the field worker you have a role to play in the process. How do you work with Angelica so that she can participate fully in this crucial decision concerning her life? It is important to consider what preparation needs to occur prior to the review, and what needs to be done during and after the review to support Angelica (Case study adapted from Coombe and Little 1986: 151.)

Commentary
Compare your ideas with those listed below. They were developed out of a training exercise designed by the authors. The participants were residential social workers who were asked to think about the issues concerning the involvement of young people in meetings.

Before the meeting
The young person needs to:

- know the purpose of the meeting;
- have the information about who will attend and why;
- have the option to request that certain people do not attend;
- be introduced to participants before the meeting;
- have had access to and understood previous minutes (e.g. child care conference notes, review notes);
- be able to go through the report to be presented at the meeting in advance (with an appropriate person);
- be aware of delicate issues that might be brought up at the meeting;
- be able to discuss how she or he might feel and react to information presented at the meeting;
- have the opportunity to participate in a 'mock' meeting if they wish;
- meet the chair of the meeting;
- feel comfortable about the timing of the meeting (i.e. not to have to miss school or work).

During the meeting

- The young person should be properly introduced to the participants of the meeting and made aware of its purpose.
- The young person should be allowed to communicate in a way that is comfortable to her or him.
- The young person should have a right to leave at any point. This is to be agreed prior to the start of the meeting and if necessary a short break in the proceedings is to be allowed.
- Participants need to be aware of the possible reactions of the young person.
- A support strategy must be developed and agreed so that it is clear who is to support the young person and how this should be managed.

• Thought should be given to the length of the meeting. This means that there should be clear aims and objectives so that only pertinent information is discussed.

After the meeting

• The young person should have the opportunity to discuss the process and the decisions taken and
   (a) be able to express any feelings that she or he may have;
   (b) be able to explore the implications of the decisions made.
• The young person should have access to support.
• The young person should receive her or his own copy of the minutes.

The following points were suggested to aid the above process

• A code of conduct needs to be sent out to all participants prior to the meeting.
• Chairs should have access to training.
• The young person should not be referred to as the 'subject' in written documentation.

This is not a complete list and you may well wish to add to it. Although they are specifically related to young people the principles can be transferred and used with other groups. These are general guidelines. In some situations it will be necessary to adapt them to meet the needs of an individual. For example, it may be that a person with learning difficulties will become very distressed by having to sit too long in one position, or may become frustrated with all the written work presented at the meeting. Guidelines about how best a service user's needs may be met should therefore be circulated to all participants.

12   EVALUATION

Evaluation of one's mental and physical state is unlikely if the
space so essential to the unhurried frame of mind is absent, so we
need to ponder the value of creating space and contemplate the
disposition generated by being in a hurry.

(Rees 1991: 121)

The essence of evaluating is to make that 'space' so that you can 'ponder'.
And why are we pondering? We are pondering in order constantly to remind
ourselves of what we are doing and why we are doing it. Our interaction
with people should make a difference to their lives and to our lives.

In this chapter we will give thought to the importance of evaluation at
practice and policy levels and what legislation tells us about evaluation. First
we will consider the process of evaluation – this will mean looking at personal evaluation as well as the use of monitoring procedures. For us it is
particularly important to think about how we are using the law and how to
improve practice. It is also about analysing where the gaps are and how to
close those gaps. We will then go on to consider how agencies have responded
to the requirements of legislation to monitor and evaluate service provision
effectively through quality assurance and inspection units. Finally, we will
look at some examples of how change can be promoted through effective
evaluation techniques.

Legislation and evaluation

More recent legislation reflects the need of the market economy to have
measurable outcomes. Within the legislation, therefore, there are in-built
objectives in relation to service delivery and effective use of resources.

Several documents have been produced as a consequence of the legislation, stating clearly the need for health and social care agencies to have explicit objectives.

- Social services authorities are expected to produce social and/or community care plans.
- Agencies have a legal duty to work together. Many authorities are working together as partners to produce corporate plans in relation to service provision where they provide services under the same pieces of legislation. In relation to services for children and families these would include: the Children Act 1989, the Education Acts 1985 and 1993, Sections 5 and 6 of the Disabled Persons' Act 1986, the NHS Community Care Act 1990, Carers (Recognition and Services) Act 1995, the Criminal Justice Act 1991, 1993, the Criminal Justice and Public Order Act 1994 and the Adoption Act 1984. Agencies working together in this respect would include: city/metropolitan borough councils; district health authorities; NHS health care trusts; family health services authorities and voluntary organizations.
- Health and local authorities are expected to develop community services to help vulnerable people to live as independently as possible in their own homes (DoH 1989; NHS and Community Care Act 1990).
- The White Paper *Health of the Nation* (DoH 1992c) sets targets for a healthier population, e.g.: to reduce the death rate for breast cancer among people invited for screening between the ages of 50 and 64 years by at least 25 per cent by the year 2000; to reduce the overall suicide rate by at least 15 per cent by the year 2000.
- The 1991 Citizen's Charter is based on the idea of public sector organizations having specific targets or objectives, e.g. health authorities in relation to waiting times. Citizens can then claim compensation where organizations fail to meet stated objectives.

The importance of ongoing evaluation

It could be said that evaluation is a tool for measuring quality. That process involves examining aims and objectives, in order to question and examine what we are doing. Having done that we are then able to contribute to decision making (i.e. by providing new information which can lead to changes) and to improve the quality of service provision. Evaluation should not just be a private enterprise – it is about opening up our work to public scrutiny. This is important if we are to be accountable for how public resources are used to meet the needs of people who require a service. Evaluation is a continuous process and should be an integral part of the way we work. It should also incorporate the views of everyone involved in the process of providing health and social care services.

Evaluation is essentially a series of procedures which are carried out in order to collect information. This will then 'improve the quality of a service' by underpinning the decision making and allow us to judge the 'quality of the services we offer' (Edwards 1991). Evaluation is often referred to as *formative* or *summative*. Formative evaluation is carried out at regular intervals and the information can be used to provide continuous feedback to inform and reshape the process. Summative evaluation is concerned with outcomes and effectiveness. Its purpose is to provide a final report about a project or programme but it will not be used for continuous reshaping.

We started off in our assessment and planning chapters with a map to chart the journey to empowerment. By taking account of all the events we are involved in we monitor our journey. Formative evaluation is about continually checking where we are going to make sure we are on the right track. When we have reached the end of the journey we provide a summative evaluation which should attempt to answer these questions:

Have we arrived at our destination?
- If 'no', where are we?
- If 'yes', or 'no', how did we arrive there?
- If 'yes', or 'no', is it worth going on? (Phillips *et al.* 1994: 4.)

Evaluation is not just something we do because we think it is a good idea! We feel it is important – but more than that, so do government departments. They recognize the need to evaluate and monitor the laws they produce and oversee as public servants. No doubt the government also has its own reasons for disseminating *certain* information about how legislation is functioning. However, we need to use their reports and statistics to inform our practice and actively to involve ourselves and service users in debate. Through this process people can be made aware of their rights and promote campaigns in order to ensure that these rights are respected.

Evaluation in practice

The service manager at Angelfields Resource Centre for Older People decided that it was important to evaluate the range of activities that the Centre was offering to the users. She decided to bring it to one of the regular user committee meetings. Before the meeting she spoke to Arthur, who was the chair of the group, and told him that the Centre was due to be inspected and that she wanted to find out whether the activities were acceptable. She was particularly proud of the Old Time Musical Evening that she personally arranged once a month. Arthur agreed to put the inspection visit on the agenda, although he pointed out that there was already a full agenda. He told her that she would have to limit her input to ten minutes.

The users had agreed that meetings would last no longer than an hour. Usually the officer in charge did not attend. However, on this occasion Arthur informed the meeting that she had especially asked to attend, to find out what the users felt about the activities offered. This did upset a few people and Arthur had to stop further discussion about the invitation. Arthur felt that this did not bode well for the rest of the meeting. It was not a good start. The service manager gave out a questionnaire which took some time to fill in. Points of clarification were brought up and some people indicated that they would have preferred more time to consider their responses. One person did not have her reading glasses to hand. The service manager then spoke for 20 minutes about the inspection. Some of those present were nodding off at this stage.

The meeting went on for two hours. Only one item was discussed, despite the fact that there was a prearranged agenda. At the end of the meeting the service manager pleased with her input, told the users that she would take the information she had obtained to the next staff meeting. This would help her evaluate the services offered. Some of the users felt the need for a stiff drink! Arthur considered that he had not managed the meeting well. He thought that inviting her to the meeting would be helpful but it turned out to be a nightmare.

In terms of the above scenario how far do you feel that the users were consulted or involved in the process of evaluation? Perhaps the following questions need to be asked.

- What was the purpose of this evaluation?
- Do you think that the service manager actually gathered the information she needed?
- Do you think that the service manager would have the correct information in order to meet the needs of the users?

The ethos of the Centre was to empower users; hence the user committee meetings.

- How far do you think that the actions of the service manager enhanced or hindered empowerment of the committee members?
- Do you feel that following the staff meeting a useful summative evaluation could be obtained?
- Do you feel that any changes recommended will actually occur?

You should now have an understanding of the importance of evaluation. But is it that simple? What is monitoring? Are monitoring and evaluation the same, different, or part and parcel of the same process? And where do quality assurance and inspection units fit in? We will now go on to look at some of these issues.

Monitoring or evaluation?

Monitoring can be defined as 'the systematic and continuous surveillance of a series of events' (Phillips *et al.* 1994: 1). Monitoring does not give a full picture on its own and needs to be a part of the process of evaluation. It is specifically concerned with procedures and processes. But it is important to combine this with evaluation procedures in order to obtain a full and sensitive analysis of a situation. For example, monitoring how well a service is reaching people of differing social divisions would give a statistical analysis of how many women, how many black people, how many disabled people or how many people with learning difficulties actually received the service.

A monitoring exercise carried out at Angelfields Resource Centre found that only a small proportion of the users actually attended the Old Time Musical Evenings. It also identified that a number of the staff would come in with their friends and families, even if they were *off duty*, to participate – the service manager thought this was a good indication of how well the community was involved in the Centre.

Monitoring can give you a snapshot of what is happening and identify groups to target. But it cannot tell you the reasons why a particular group is not receiving the service. Thus it will provide a database for policy decisions and judgements regarding quality and efficiency. It requires a set of judgements about what to monitor but does not include criteria for making policy decisions (Edwards 1991).

Inspections

The Social Services Inspectorate defines inspection as 'a process of quality control which itself is only part of a wider management system aimed at ensuring the quality of care provided and the quality of life for users' (Wing 1991: i). The NHS and Community Care Act 1990 and the Children Act 1989 have changed the role and function of inspection and quality control quite dramatically in health and social care practice. *Arm's length* inspection units have been set up within social services departments and health care services are inspected through the Health Advisory Service. Inspection should now be an enabling process, which does not just identify shortfalls in standards, but also points the way towards improving practice. It needs to take account not only of how services are managed, but also of what structures exist to enable users to exercise a greater degree of choice. The change in focus can perhaps be demonstrated by the inclusion of *user consultants* in inspections of children's homes. The Social Services Inspectorate, in 1992, introduced the idea of involving young people who had experienced care as part of inspection teams. They involved young people in this way because they saw it as a means of incorporating a user perspective into the inspection process. The whole inspection team would work to the same agenda but the younger members of the team focused on different aspects of care. As one young inspector explained:

> We are very hot on children's rights, clothing allowances, choice of food, sanctions, complaints and what the staff write about the children. Past users look at it from a child centred point of view and are less interested in managerial structures.
>
> (*Community Care*, 2 December 1993)

It has been said that inspections have limitations in terms of evaluating quality of care (Phillips *et al.* 1994). The number of inspections per inspector is too high to allow close monitoring. There is inevitably a lack of independence even for long arm inspection units, as inspectors are employed by the authority they are inspecting. An independent element can be incorporated if users and carers are partners in the process. But, at the time of writing, the regular involvement of users and carers in inspection teams is not common practice.

Everitt *et al.* (1992: 124) note that monitoring and arm's length inspection units are 'both top down mechanisms to check on the implementation of and adherence to standards in practice'. They point out that the methodology used to collect data does not necessarily allow for bad practice to be identified. Enquiries concerning abuse of young people in residential homes, for instance, demonstrates that 'more qualitative and subjective data on performance will be collected and examined only when something goes wrong – and then in an inquisitorial context' (Everitt *et al.* 1992: 124).

Ironing out the contradictions

Evaluation has been said to be a 'revolutionary activity' (Phillips *et al.* 1994: 24). Since the emphasis for health and social care practitioners is now focused on user involvement and empowerment of service users, effective evaluation is essential. What do we mean by this revolutionary activity?

> The concept of user empowerment, in the name of which many new schemes are being set up and evaluated, is breathtakingly radical in its implications for shifts of power and influence in service planning and modes of service provision.
>
> (Phillips *et al.* 1994: 24)

Such a revolutionary change took place when Angelfields Resource Centre, established to provide a range of services for older people, was evaluated. The service was set up by professionals, who identified the need for a range of services to meet the needs of older people in varying circumstances. The staff team genuinely wanted to empower the people with whom they were working and ensure that their voices were heard. After three years the service was evaluated by an independent consultant. In the course of her evaluation the consultant interviewed a selection of people, including members of the staff team, the management group and service users. The outcome of her evaluation was that, although the service was well used and respected by both professionals and service users, it had not incorporated a users' perspective. She wrote in her concluding remarks:

> *There has been a singular lack of consultation with users and thus the power of the professionals has never been challenged. This does not deny the very real contribution of committed professionals who have worked hard to set up the service. But it is a salutary reminder of the difficulty professionals have in truly sharing power. For the service to move on there is a need for the professionals to understand what user involvement and working in partnership really means. This means that power must be shared with the users – which must inevitably mean a loss of power by professionals.*

That information was then used as a basis to revise the service and address practice issues.

The legislation expects users to participate in decisions made about their own lives at a personal level, as well as being involved at the structural level of policy and planning. Without proper evaluation of personal practice, of the impact of the legislation and the policies and procedures that derive from that, it can be easy to delude ourselves into believing that a commitment to user involvement means that it is actually happening.

Can we as practitioners and carers really have any influence?

Everitt *et al.* note that practitioner evaluation is essential. They express the hope that the new systems of quality control and inspection units will become part and parcel of the routine of health and social welfare organizations.

Currently, as they point out, it is often 'left to brave practitioners and brave users to comment on bad practice. To ensure that quality systems really work they need to be empowered' (Everitt *et al*. 1992: 125).

There are many opportunities for us to be involved in the evaluation of our work. However, these may not seem immediately obvious. There are the inspections we have already talked about, which are there for us to contribute to. Quality assurance units have also been set up to monitor, evaluate and develop practice. Conferences and research projects, either independently funded or funded through government resources, can yield significant information about practice and how the legislation is being used. These are available for carers and health and social care practitioners to attend, or contribute to. The government also publishes reports and consultation papers which provide both information and the opportunity to comment on various aspects of legislation.

Let us look at some opportunities that have been documented concerning legislation for children and its implementation.

Regional conference for guardians ad litem *and reporting officers*

Between June and October 1993 the Department of Health jointly sponsored with IRCHIN (Independent Representation for Children in Need) a series of four regional conferences for guardians *ad litem* and reporting officers. The four reports produced reflected the regional response, focusing on one of a number of areas. We will look at one of the areas, which was that of *contact* between children and young people and significant people in their lives. In relation to how contact arrangements are worked out it was clear from the workshop reports that this was an area of concern.

Despite the fact that it is a central tenet of the Act, the issue of contact between children and families is seen by practitioners to be characterized by inconsistency and a low priority in terms of consideration of contact as a part of care plans. Participants reported that there appeared to be no regard for the effects that this might have on individual children, and the need for a child-centred approach was highlighted in the reports. Contact is supposed to be looked at and positively promoted, taking into account the wishes and feelings of children and their cultural needs. It was noted in one report that courts have overruled the local authority in contact matters and determined the case on the needs of the individual child.

Good anti-oppressive practice is about taking account of this evidence of practice, measuring it against the requirements of the legislation and then measuring the discrepancy. For carers and practitioners it is about ensuring that contact is central to care plans and considers the needs of the child. For guardians *ad litem*, who are in the privileged position of advising the courts, it may therefore mean asking the courts to override local authority decisions in contact matters. Therefore, the evaluation provided through the conference reports gives practitioners the evidence which they can then use to develop good practice, provide relevant training opportunities and promote change within the legislative framework. For the conference organizers the views and experience of the 425 guardians *ad litem* provided 'an impressive and

informative body of information about current panel practice and the developments which have taken place in the service following implementation of
the Children Act 1989' (Timms 1993: 2).

Reassessing priorities: CHAR research project

Young people are a powerless and marginalized group in our society. Oppression of young people is highlighted by the fact that recently young people
have been adversely affected by legislation in a number of areas, such as
education, social security and housing. Young people who are also homeless
face even more discrimination. The Children Act 1989 was therefore seen by
many agencies working with young homeless people as providing them with
a greater opportunity to receive housing and support services from local
authorities.

In July 1993, CHAR, the housing campaign for single people, produced a
report, funded by the Nuffield Foundation, which was the first stage of a
two-year research project. The aim of the research was to carry out a comprehensive national assessment of how the Children Act was being implemented to meet the needs of young homeless people. However, the research
findings uncovered the fact that many local authorities are disregarding the
legislation in this area and in some cases 'blatantly contravening' the law.
The report made a number of recommendations and some in particular in
relation to the legislation.

- The legislation should be clarified and additional guidance issued, thus
  identifying social services departments' responsibility to homeless 16- and
  17-year-olds. Within the legislation, many powers should become duties,
  particularly those parts of the Act which cover leaving care arrangements.
- Guidance and clarification of the Act is required in relation to young
  homeless people, particularly with regard to: Section 27 of the Children
  Act, as it relates to Part III of the Housing Act 1985, especially *vis à vis*
  unitary authorities; and Section 24, the leaving care aspects of the Children Act.
- With the aim of assisting the assessments of young homeless people, the
  government should amend the guidance of Part III of the Housing Act
  1985 to ensure that the definition of 'vulnerability' includes all homeless
  16- and 17-year-olds, and to bring it into line with the definition of 'child
  in need whose welfare is seriously prejudiced' under the Children Act 1989.

This provides CHAR and other campaigning organizations with the evidence
to lobby MPs in an attempt to bring about the relevant changes. It also
provides workers in social service and housing departments with material to
consider their practice in this area and use the law to reduce, or even elim-
inate, homelessness among young people.

The Children Act Advisory Committee

Government itself sets up bodies to monitor legislation. The Children Act
Advisory Committee was therefore set up, before the Act received Royal

Assent, to monitor its operation and implementation. The terms of reference were:

> To advise the Lord Chancellor, the Home Secretary, the Secretary of State for Health and the President of the Family Division on whether the guiding principles of the Children Act 1989 are being achieved and whether the court procedures and the guardian ad litem system are operating satisfactorily.
>
> (Children Act Advisory Committee 1991/2)

These terms of reference were reviewed after two years and were changed to make them less limiting:

> To advise . . . on the progress of the Children Act cases through the court system, with a view to identifying special difficulties and reducing avoidable delay.
>
> To promote through local Family Court Business Committees commonality of administrative practice and procedure in the Family Proceedings Courts and the County Courts, and to advise on the impact Children Act work of other family initiatives.
>
> (Children Act Advisory Committee 1992/3)

In the second annual report the Committee:

- makes observations with regard to ongoing monitoring;
- comments about good practice;
- comments about bad practice;
- notes matters to be brought to the attention of ministers.

In relation to the Court Welfare Service, for example, the report notes that there have been significant delays in the production of reports – which was felt to be unsatisfactory. The Committee therefore arranged to monitor the national situation by regular updates from the Family Court Business Committees. It is also keeping 'under review' (Children Act Advisory Committee 1992/3: 27) delays in setting dates for private law cases.

In other instances the Committee invites comments on certain situations; for example, in procedures for urgent applications in the High Court the 'Committee notes with approval the existing arrangements. It invites comment on their use, possible improvements or difficulties encountered' (Children Act Advisory Committee 1992/3: 69). Similarly, it invites comments on 'the sorts of difficulties that have arisen in practice' (Children Act Advisory Committee 1992/3: 19) in the interrelationship of concurrent civil and criminal proceedings. In this way ongoing monitoring of the situation from practitioners is encouraged.

In terms of noting how practice might be improved, the Committee makes various comments. For example, in relation to the use of interim care orders the Committee makes a strong statement about the improper use of such orders. It appears that courts have used interim orders as a means of keeping a case under review as they lack confidence in the local authority's ability to carry out care plans. More strongly still, the Committee states that it will think about making representations to ministers about providing courts with the power to make a short-term emergency ouster order to remove an abuser or suspected abuser from the home.

Clearly, the ongoing monitoring of the Act in this way can only assist practitioners in ensuring that the legislation is not oppressive to children, young people and their families. It provides information about the current situation and observations about practice issues and the implementation of the law, and gives practitioners the opportunity to comment on their experiences of the legislation in practice. It is the responsibility of all those engaged in health and social care practice to read reports that may exist in their field of work, and to take the opportunities provided to feed into the forums which can influence practice guidance papers and possible changes in the law. The reports may reflect government bias but this is not a reason to ignore them – rather, they should be read in the light of your own knowledge and understanding of the issues. While changing the law is not easy, it is only by constantly bringing issues to the attention of those who can effect change that there will be any movement forward.

Data collection

Data collection and the monitoring of trends is an important aspect of evaluation in respect of legislation. For example, the Children Act 1989 introduced a number of changes, including the following:

- avoiding the use of courts in family matters;
- reducing delay in proceedings;
- ascertaining the wishes and feelings of children.

A research study undertaken for a conference organized by the Humberside Court Welfare Service in November 1992 found that the Act has not reduced the number of referrals to the court welfare service. Divorced fathers are becoming less involved in the legal processes but other groups, such as grandparents, are becoming more involved. Delay in the production of reports has significantly reduced and involving children and young people is now on the agenda.

The Humberside survey highlighted a number of issues, not only concerning the importance of data collection but also about the need for ongoing debate about service development. It noted that 'changing the law without providing the mediation and conciliation services to support families will do little to achieve the Act's objective of reducing the courts' role to a place of last resort' (Trinder 1993: 484). Practitioners and carers therefore need to know about research findings in their particular area of work, and use them in evaluation of their own services, in order to provide an effective service to meet people's needs.

Final thoughts

Many of us within the health and social services do not allow ourselves the time to 'ponder'. The pressures of work are such that finding the space to read, reflect and evaluate our practice can be difficult. In a society where policies are shaped by dominant values and norms little account is taken of the needs of oppressed groups. Recent legislation has started to address the needs of some oppressed groups although we know that others are still specifically oppressed by particular legislation or lack of it. It is therefore essential to monitor and evaluate the effectiveness of all legislation by making ourselves aware of relevant research and law reports.

Within our practice it is important to be aware of the 'evidence of inequities, inequalities and problems of accessibility' which 'abound at all levels, within and across societies' (Phillips *et al.* 1994: 163). If we are to ensure that our practice does not further disempower we need to evaluate constantly what we are doing and why we are doing it. At the heart of evaluation is *change*, and effective evaluative techniques can promote change.

> Evaluation becomes concerned with making visible what goes on in practice. Its purpose is not simply to test whether narrowly defined objectives have been met. It is continually to question and problematise definitions of social need and established responses to that need. Further it is to understand and make explicit the impact of economies and social policies and structures on the chances of practice moving in the direction of the 'good'.
>
> (Everitt *et al.* 1992: 130)

Activities

Activity 1

We all have the capacity to evaluate our own situation. It might be at an individual level, a team level or an organizational level. You may be nursing on a large medical ward, caring for a dependent relative, working in a small voluntary organization or part of a social work team. This exercise is intended to help you to evaluate your own practice and identify whether you are providing a quality service.

To begin, use the following questions in relation to your own situation:

1 Clearly define your aims and objectives.
   (a) What is it that you really want to achieve?
   (b) What obstacles stand in the way of your task?
   (c) What do you need to do to overcome the obstacles?
   (d) What will the reward be?
   (e) Is the task worth the reward?
2 Think about your answers and evaluate them.
   (a) Are your aims and objectives realistic?
   (b) Can they be achieved in the time available?
   (c) Are they appropriate (to the family, your agency, yourself)?
   (d) Are they compatible with policies, guidelines, procedures, legislation?
   (e) Are they in the best interests of the service user?
   (f) Are they measurable?

Activity 2

The community care legislation has an impact on agency policy and practice. This exercise can be used to assist in evaluating the planning and delivery of community care services. Can you answer the questions in respect of your own situation?

1 What groups or sub-groups is the organization seeking to help (for example older people or people with mental health problems)?
2 What specific needs do the groups have? What problems are the organization's services aimed at reducing?
3 Who is identifying and defining the needs and/or problems? The target groups themselves? Their formal carers? Clients' advocates? Professionals? Some combination of these?
4 How are the needs to be identified? How are the assessments to be done? What procedures and documentation are to be used? (Questions adapted from Palfrey *et al.* 1990: 15.)

As part of the process of evaluation you need to think about how it will be used and who should have access to it. There will be some recommendations from the evaluation. You therefore also need to think about their implementation.

Activity 3

Evaluating inequalities in health and social care service provision is a difficult process. The following case study (taken from Phillips *et al.* 1994) highlights the dilemmas and difficulties.

GP practice accommodation
A GP practice has to find new accommodation because the current practice is located in a converted house which is part of the estate of the recently deceased senior partner.

A large new private housing estate has land allocated for a new health centre and, because demographic trends do not warrant the establishment of another practice, the Family Health Service Association (FHSA) has approved plans for the practice to move to this purpose-built accommodation. The estate has a range of houses, from one-bedroom starter homes to large executive houses, which are increasing in proportion because they are still relatively attractive despite the depressed housing market.

The community where the practice has been located for many years is an area with an ageing population living in private housing, the vast majority of the stock being at least 30 years old. Nearby is an area consisting of a mixture of council houses, housing association property and ex-council houses, where the level of unemployment is relatively high, the incidence of crime and vandalism is increasing and there are a few community homes for patients discharged from a mental hospital scheduled for closure.

1 What are the implications for accessibility to the new practice and what are the likely consequences for health inequalities between groups in the locality?
2 In what way can the FHSA offset these problems?

Commentary
Phillips *et al.* (1994) make the following observations.

1 Accessibility for the community where the practice has been located is considerably reduced.
2 It is likely that the health inequalities between different groups will be increased, unless arrangements can be made to offset the consequences of relocation.
3 What are the public transport facilities? The FHSA could minimize the transport problems caused by relocation, either by ensuring that adequate public transport is provided or by providing its own transport.
4 The FHSA could negotiate with the district health authority to provide a branch surgery in one of the community homes.
5 It could be that a more efficient service is considered to be adequate compensation for reduction in accessibility and increase in inequalities.

Think about the principles of anti-oppressive practice as you consider the dilemmas posed by the final question.

13 THE REALITY OF

ANTI-OPPRESSIVE PRACTICE

Working from an anti-oppressive position brings with it a fundamental transformation not only on an individual level but also on an organisational level. Implications for practice are expressed by Micheline Mason, one of the founder members of the Liberation Network of People with Disabilities, who says of professional intervention:

> It will involve looking at your fears about disability, and exploring your own feelings of being oppressed. It will involve giving over information which you, as professionals, have been given and which we need. It will involve practical support for initiatives which we take, and will involve redesigning your role as 'helper' into one of enabler. Most of all it will involve making friends with us on our own terms. This may feel painful, frightening, difficult or even humiliating to you, as it does to us, but we are certain that it is necessary for all of us to get through this period of fundamental change in order to live together and enjoy each other as equals.
>
> (Campling 1984: 25)

Theory, the law and practice

In the process of writing this book we have had to be constantly aware of the differences between us. But an awareness of differences is not enough – there has to be a common understanding of each other's value base. An awareness of values enables us to look at the points of contact and differences between us. What brings us together is a commitment to change and the 'sense of outrage' (Simey 1993) which introduces the book. The sense of outrage comes from our experiences and from constantly questioning what is happening in the world we live in.

Part of that commitment to change is about being prepared to change ourselves. Change involves reflecting, challenging and rethinking our taken-for-granted views of the structures within which we operate. We both have had to think carefully about the legislation, for example: because it *isn't* anti-racist, it *isn't* anti-sexist and in some cases it *is* discriminatory.

Throughout this book we have constantly referred to the need to be aware of and understand your own value base, as well as to understand that this might be different from the prevailing ideology. In our own work we are aware of what our value base is. That is not to say that we are not prepared to change – far from it. We have changed as we have explored issues. We have challenged each other, and in that process have inevitably changed and developed our knowledge of our own value bases. Essentially this process of change is the core of anti-oppressive practice.

We have chosen the law to demonstrate that it is possible to promote change and that legislation can be used as a tool for anti-oppressive practice. We see the law as a powerful force. That power can be problematic in that it can be oppressive, but it can be used to empower people who are marginalized within society. We identify and take the positive aspects of the law that fit our value base and ideology and use them to support anti-oppressive practice.

We recognize and acknowledge that oppression and inequality exist within society and are reflected in service provision. The existence of legislation provides for us 'a framework within which concerns can be raised and details of procedure and practice discussed' (Connelly 1989: 30). In terms of anti-oppressive practice we feel that this provides one of the few arenas to put issues on the agenda for debate. It is only through open discussion that we are able to reflect on attitudes and beliefs and exploit the opportunities presented to us within legislation to combat oppression and oppressive practices.

Consistency in our practice arises from a desire for change informed by an understanding of power and powerlessness, the experiences of people who have been oppressed and marginalized and our own experiences of oppression, powerlessness and being in powerful positions. Our viewpoint is also informed by others who have written about their experiences – their personal biographies – by documented research evidence, by the richness of cultures expressed through poetry, literature and drama. This is important because 'sharing ideas from various sources to express the relationship between personal context and the dominant values in a culture represents the promise of biography' (Rees 1991: 10). It is through the telling of our stories that the complexities of life are highlighted (Harris and Timms 1993a). The process of making links between our personal biographies and the structures of society is of itself empowering.

There are two elements which inform our anti-oppressive practice: the dual perspective and the process of empowerment. An understanding of the dual perspective helps us to understand the position of oppressed people – not just by reference to themselves but also by reference to the wider society. In considering the principles in Part II and the practice in Part III we have consistently tried to make the links between the personal and the structural. By understanding both the structure and people's personal biographies we have a 'rich explanation of the interactive process of change' (Juckes and Barresi 1993: 214). So what do we think anti-oppressive practice is? Reflect on the following statement.

> I tried to disappear into myself in order to deflect the painful, daily assaults designed to teach me that being an African-American, working class woman made me lesser than those who were not. And as I felt smaller, I became quieter and eventually was virtually silenced.
>
> (Hill-Collins 1990: xi)

This conveys for us very forcefully why anti-oppressive practice is so important. Anti-oppressive practice is about making sure that people are never silenced. How do we do this? We offer for consideration the following pointers or critical triggers (Ahmed 1994) which inform our practice:

- we challenge the use of power;
- we question the way things are, e.g. poverty, unemployment, sexism, racism, homophobia;
- we believe that people should define their own oppression;
- we have a commitment to change – part of that commitment is making visible people's stories and, having done that, we try to work with them to start to make the links and so find a way forward;
- we have an understanding and knowledge of the legislation;
- we use the legislation positively to facilitate change;
- we challenge oppressive legislation;
- we look at how we use legislation to inform our practice;
- we look at the gaps to see how we can improve the legislation that is there;
- we work in partnership and involve users;
- we believe in the concept of minimal intervention;
- we constantly evaluate as part of our practice;
- we endeavour to communicate effectively;
- we look at what we have in common with users, carers, colleagues and other workers and we see any differences as a basis for discussion, to widen our understanding rather than limit us;
- we try to address the international links and how they affect our practice and the people we work with.

The purpose of this book is to enable practitioners and carers to make the links between issues of power and oppression that lie at the heart of health and social care practice. We have attempted to develop a practice which addresses power imbalances by using the powerful structure of the law to achieve change. We therefore need to conclude by thinking about that process of change.

First, it is important to remember why change might be necessary. Change is necessary if we recognize the 'complexity and diversity of the manifold oppressions that affect the lives' (Langan 1992: 1) of all of us. Equality, equity and accessibility have been identified as vital social and political goals in the delivery of health and social care services (Phillips *et al.* 1994). There are many ways of attempting to achieve these goals. However, there are divergent opinions as to how to do so, affected by different theoretical approaches and understandings of oppression within society. Our argument, using the dual perspective, is that change is only possible through an understanding of the link between the personal and the structural inequalities that exist.

There has been an attempt within social care practice to address these issues. But change is not easy and can have both financial and personal costs. Lack of resources characterizes the delivery of health and social care services. For example, Twigg and Atkin (1994: 64) found in their research focusing on carers that in relation to the work of occupational therapists 'the realities of their day-to-day work, in the context of waiting lists and backlogs, means that practice is much more narrowly focused'. To widen the focus in all areas of practice requires a commitment to challenging inequalities. Rooney (1987) identified strong resistance to change from central and local government in relation to avoidance of the financial costs of that change. This means that the personal costs to practitioners and carers in fighting for change are directly related to fighting for increased resources as well as having to fight the ideological battles. However, as Rooney (1987: 97) points out, 'Where change did come about it was through the ability to find and use power, no great measure of it but little bits here and there.' We have said the law is a powerful resource. If we can use that power as an opportunity system (Solomon 1976), even 'little bits here and there', then we can promote change.

Short-term and long-term strategies

In a busy week, with few resources, you may feel that it is unrealistic even to consider strategies for promoting change – it is all you can do to keep things going! However, we are not talking about changing the world overnight, we are talking about informing our practice: small changes are as important as major changes. Obviously, *campaigning* for major changes, such as legislation to outlaw discrimination against people with disabilities or supporting campaigns to promote equality for lesbian and gay people, is crucial. At the same time, it is necessary to beware of the popular press playing on ignorance and fear and creating a backlash which may not be helpful. Equally important, therefore, is our *practice* in working with people with disabilities and gay men and lesbians. The available legislation for these groups of people is oppressive, but there is legislation that can be used to promote anti-oppressive practice.

To combat oppression and empower individuals it is helpful to develop a strategy for change. A strategy can be defined as the development of a plan of action which goes beyond a passive commitment to anti-oppressive principles. It is the development of specific goals and timetables for the achievement of equality. This can only be achieved if you first consider: the *opposing forces*, i.e. the oppressive climate; and the *supporting forces*, i.e. legislation, opportunities and commitment. There is a process that involves looking at the terrain. Other people have travelled these paths before: so you need to acknowledge this and inform yourself. The following points then need to be considered when you are thinking about strategies.

You need to identify the issue, problem or goal

Consider the following statistics. Sixty per cent of people over the age of 70 in residential and nursing homes have impaired hearing. Fewer than one-quarter have hearing aids (*Community Care*, 15 April 1993). What impact does this have on you? What does this tell us about practice with older people in society? What does this tell us about how we perceive the rights of older people? If we know these facts what are we doing about them? The voluntary organization Counsel and Care has suggested that community care reforms are unlikely to make any difference. However, at the heart of community care legislation is the provision of better services for those who need them. Good practice in this case must be about using the available legislation to make a difference, change that statistic and improve the quality of life and empower older people with impaired hearing. The specific issue in this case could be identified as impaired hearing. The goal could be to improve the quality of life for older people in residential care. Alternatively there could be other policy and practice issues.

Break down the issue, problem or goal so that it is manageable

Assessments should take account of any hearing difficulty, and once stated the care plan should include whether a hearing test has been provided and what action is taken given the results of the test.

Set a time limit or target (this is dependent on the task)

Counsel and Care recommends that care staff could be trained to fit and adjust hearing aids. The home as part of its admissions procedure could ensure that a hearing test is offered to all residents, and care plans could specify action to be taken. The targets could be:

- staff training;
- negotiating for resources;
- reviewing practices and procedures;
- developing policies.

Review and evaluate

Some examples of what could be included are:

- Has a record been kept of how many staff have been trained?
- Have any additional training needs been identified?
- Have adequate resources been obtained (it is no use having a box of hearing aids with no batteries)?
- Do all staff know the admissions policy?

Make links with others

There is always resistance to change. Staff will therefore need support within individual residential establishments but can also make links with others in relation to training, reviewing practices and procedures and developing new policies.

It is important to develop practice which incorporates such strategies but we must be sure not to simplify the issue and to remember that oppression is complex. It has to be tackled at both the *personal* and the *structural* levels and solutions might not always be straightforward. We can often tackle the practical concrete elements of a problem but it is more difficult to challenge the ideologies which maintain oppressive practices.

Ideological change incorporates an understanding of the linkages and interconnections between various oppressions. However, it is a lot more difficult to promote such change. It is necessary for ideological and concrete change to go hand in hand if any effective permanent change is to occur.

It is easy to be 'overwhelmed by the sheer scale and range of issues' (Lynn 1991: 13) in relation to anti-oppressive practice. In discussing empowerment we put forward a model for practice which enables us to understand that oppression operates at a number of levels. The benefit of working from such a model is that it enables you to think about how, and at which level, work needs to be undertaken.

Final thoughts

If we are committed to anti-oppressive practice then we have a duty to ensure that the rights of users are not violated. Legislation can be used to deny rights but we need to be aware of our role in minimizing the oppressive aspects of practice and the law and we must endeavour to maximize the rights to which all people are entitled. It is for this reason that we see the law as an instrument to protect people's rights. It is a powerful instrument but it is one that we can control and we should not therefore become subservient to it. The following statement sums up how we should view the law in relation to our practice:

> It is up to practitioners to utilize the law in the improvement of practice. It is there. It is a gift. Use it. By setting precedents, case law will improve our practice. Leave it to the policy makers to curtail our action. Don't limit ourselves. Use the arena or platform of the law for change.
> (Paul Wilcox, project manager 1994)

BIBLIOGRAPHY

Aaron, J. and Walby, S. (1991) *Out of the Margins: Women Studies in the Nineties*. London: The Falmer Press.

Adams, R. (1990) *Self-help Social Work and Empowerment*. London: BASW/Macmillan.

Ahmad, B. (1990) *Black Perspectives in Social Work*. Birmingham: Venture Press.

Ahmed, S., Cheetham, J. and Small, J. (eds) (1986) *Social Work with Black Children and Their Families*. London: Batsford.

Anderson, S. (1993) Unpublished lecture, Liverpool John Moores University.

Andrews, G. (ed.) (1991) *Citizenship*. London: Lawrence and Wishart.

Arnstein, S. (1969) A ladder of citizen participation. *Journal of American Institute and Planners*, **35**(4), 216–24.

Aspen (1983) For my apolitical sisters, in *The Raving Beauties in the Pink*. London: The Women's Press.

Bamford, F. N. and Wolkind, S. N. (1988) *The Physical and Mental Health of Children in Care*. London: ESRC.

Bandura, A. (1982) Self-efficacy mechanism in human agency. *American Psychologist*, **37**, 122–7.

Barclay Report (1982) *Social Workers: Their Role and Tasks*. London: Bedford Square Press.

Barford, R. and Wattam, C. (1991) Children's participation in Decision Making. *Practice*, **5**(2), 93–102.

Barker, R. and Roberts, H. (1992) The uses of the concept of power, in D. Morgan and L. Stanley (eds) *Debates in Sociology*, pp. 195–224. Manchester: Manchester University Press.

Barn, R. (1983) *Black Children in the Public Care System*. London: Batsford.

Bell, M. (1993) See no evil, speak no evil, hear no evil. *Community Care Inside*, 28 October.

Bereano, N. K. (1984) Introduction, in A. Lorde, *Sister Outsider: Essays and Speeches*, CA 95019: The Crossing Press/Freedom.

Beresford, P. and Croft, S. (1993) *Citizen Involvement: a Practical Guide for Change*. London: Macmillan.

Berridge, D. (1985) *Children's Homes*. Oxford: Blackwell.

Beveridge Report (1942) *Social Insurance and the Allied Services*. London: HMSO.

Biestek, F. P. (1961) *The Casework Relationship*. London: George Allen and Unwin.

Bond, R. A. and Lemon, N. F. (1979) Changes in magistrates during the first years on the bench, in S. Lloyd Bostock (ed.) *Psychology, Law and Legal Processes.* London: Macmillan.

Booth, T. and Booth, W. (1994) *Parenting Under Pressure: Mothers and Fathers with Learning Difficulties.* Buckingham: Open University Press.

Bornat, J., Pereira, C., Pilgrim, D. and Williams, M. (eds) (1993) *Anthology: Charter in Community Care. A Reader.* London: Macmillan/Open University.

Bradshaw, J. (1972) The concept of social need. *New Society,* **3**(3–72), 640–3.

Bradshaw, J., Clifton, M. and Kennedy, J. (1978) Found dead, in A. Tinker (ed.) *The Elderly in Modern Society,* 2nd edn. London: Longman.

Brandon, A. and Brandon, D. (1987) *Consumers as Colleagues.* London: Mind Publications.

Brandon, D. and Brandon, A. (1988) *Putting People First: a Handbook on the Practical Application of Ordinary Living Principles.* London: Good Impressions Publishing.

Braye, S. and Preston-Shoot, M. (1992a) *Practising Social Work.* London: Macmillan.

Braye, S. and Preston-Shoot, M. (1992b) Honourable intentions: partnership and written agreement in welfare legislation. *Journal of Social Welfare and Family Law,* **6**, 511–28.

Braye, S. and Preston-Shoot, M. (1993) Partnership practice: responding to the challenge, realising the potential. *Social Work Education,* **12**(2), 35–53.

Brayne, H. and Martin, G. (1990) *Law for Social Workers.* London: Blackstone Press.

Bryan, W. (1990) Empowering the consumer. *Children and Society,* **4**(1), 114–19.

Burke, B. (1990) Black women want to be heard: a study of the experiences of black women social workers employed in the Liverpool Social Services Department. Unpublished MA thesis. University of Liverpool.

Burke, B. and Dalrymple, J. (1991) Implementing race and culture issues using the Children Act 1989. *Panel News,* **4**(3), 4–15.

Campling, J. (1984) On our own terms. *Community Care,* 5 April, 25–6.

Carroll, L. (1865) *Alice's Adventures in Wonderland.* London: J. M. Dent & Sons.

Carter, A. (1988) *The Politics of Women's Rights.* London: Longman.

Carter, P., Jeffs, T. and Smith, M. K. (eds) (1992) *Changing Social Work and Welfare.* Buckingham: Open University Press.

Central Council for Education and Training in Social Work (1991) *DipSW Rules and Regulations for the Diploma in Social Work.* Paper 30, 2nd edn. London: CCETSW.

Cemlyn, S. (1993) Travelling in a new direction. *Community Care,* 29 April.

Chestang, L. (1972) *Character Development in a Hostile Environment.* Chicago: University of Chicago Press.

Children Act Advisory Committee (1991/2) *Annual Report.* London: HMSO.

Children Act Advisory Committee (1992/3) *Annual Report.* London: HMSO.

Children's Rights Development Unit (CRDU) (1992) Working with young people on CRDU conference. *Childright,* **95**, 18–19.

Chorcora, M. N., Jennings, E. and Lardan, N. (1994) Issues of empowerment: anti-oppressive groupwork by disabled people in Ireland. *Groupwork,* **7**(1), 63–78.

Clark, S. (1993) Bleak housing prospects. *Community Care,* 21 October.

Clifford, D. (1994) Towards an anti-oppressive social work assessment method. *Practice,* **6**(3), 226–38.

Cohen, P. (1993) A matter of judgement. *Community Care,* 10 June.

Collins, S. and Stein, M. (1989) Users fight back: collectives in social work, in C. Rojek, G. Peacock and S. Collins (eds) *The Haunt of Misery.* London: Routledge.

Common, R. and Flynn, N. (1992) What's in the contract? *Community Care*, 6 August.

Connelly, N. (1989) *Race and Change in Social Services Departments*. London: Policy Studies Institute.

Conway, M. (1979) *Rise Gonna Rise*. New York: Anchor.

Coombe, V. and Little, A. (1986) *Race and Social Work*. London: Tavistock.

Cooper, D. (1993) The Citizen's Charter and radical democracy: empowerment and exclusion within citizenship discourse. *Social and Legal Studies*, **2**, 149–71.

Coote, A. (1992) Charter blight. *Social Work Today*, 12 November, 14–15.

Cornwell, N. (1992) Assessment and accountability in community care. *Critical Social Policy*, **36**, 40–52.

Coulshed, V. (1988) *Social Work Practice: an Introduction*. London: Macmillan.

Counsel and Care (1993) The right to take risks. *Community Care*, 15 April.

Croft, S. and Beresford, P. (1989) User involvement, citizenship and social policy. *Critical Social Policy*, **26**, 5–18.

Croft, S. and Beresford, P. (1990) *From Paternalism to Participation. Involving People in Social Services*. London: Open Services Project and Joseph Rowntree Foundation.

Croft, S. and Beresford, P. (1992) The politics of participation. *Critical Social Policy*, **35**, 20–44.

Croft, S. and Beresford, P. (1993) *Citizen Involvement: a Practical Guide for Change*. London: Macmillan.

Dalley, G. (1983) Ideologies of care: a feminist contribution to the debate. *Critical Social Policy*, **8**, 72–81.

Darlow, J. (1992) *Manchester City Council v S (1991) 2 FLR 370. Family Law*, **22**, January, 16–17.

Department of Health (1988) *Protecting Children: a Guide for Social Workers Undertaking a Comprehensive Assessment*. London: HMSO.

Department of Health (1989) *Caring for People: Community Care in the Next Decade and Beyond*. London: HMSO.

Department of Health (1990) *Code of Practice: Section 118 Mental Health Act 1983*. London: HMSO.

Department of Health (1991a) *Working Together under the Children Act 1989: a Guide to Arrangements for Inter-agency Co-operation for the Protection of Children from Abuse*. London: HMSO.

Department of Health (1991b) *Care Management and Assessment: Practitioners Guide*. London: HMSO.

Department of Health (1991c) *The Children Act 1989: Guide and Regulations Volume 3, Family Placements*. London: HMSO.

Department of Health (1992a) *Circular 92(18)*. London: HMSO.

Department of Health (1992b) *Health of the Nation*, White Paper. London: HMSO.

Department of Health (1994) *National Inspection of Services to Disabled Children and Their Families*. London: HMSO.

Department of Health and Social Security (1981) *Growing Older*. London: HMSO.

Department of Health and the Welsh Office (1992) *National Standards for the Supervision of Offenders in the Community*. London: Home Office Probation Service Division.

Dolphin Project (1993) *Answering Back: Report by Young People Being Looked After on the Children Act 1989*. Southampton: CEDR, University of Southampton.

Douglas, G. (1992) *B v B (Grandparents: Residence Order). Family Law*, November.

Doyal, L. and Gough, I. (1991) *A Theory of Human Need*. London: Macmillan.

DuBois, B. and Krogsrud Miley, K. (1992) *Social Work, an Empowering Profession.* Boston: Allyn and Bacon.

Eastman, M. (1993a) Fighting it right. *Community Care,* 6 May.

Eastman, M. (1993b) Where do you draw the line? *Community Care,* 20 May.

Edwards, J. (1991) *Evaluation in Adult and Further Education.* Liverpool: WEA.

Edwards, S. and Halpern, A. (1992) Parental responsibility: an instrument of social policy. *Family Law,* March.

Ely, P. and Denney, D. (1987) *Social Work in a Multi Racial Society.* Aldershot: Gower.

Everitt, A., Hardiker, P., Littlewood, J. and Mullender, A. (1992) *Applied Research for Better Practice.* London: Macmillan.

Fallon, S. (1992) Turning the tide. *Community Care,* 26 March.

Feinberg, J. (1966) Duties, rights and claims. *American Philosophical Quarterly,* **2**(3), 1.

Fennell, G., Phillipson, C. and Evers, H. (1988) *The Sociology of Old Age.* Milton Keynes: Open University Press.

Fennell, P. (1989) Falling through the legal loopholes. *Social Work Today,* 30 November, 18–20.

Finch, J. (1989) *Family Obligations and Social Change.* Cambridge: Polity Press.

Finch, J. and Groves, D. (1980) Community care and the family: a case for equal opportunities. *Journal of Social Policy,* **9**(4), 487–514.

Finch, J. and Mason, J. (1990) *Negotiating Family Responsibility.* London: Routledge.

Fox-Harding, L. (1991) *Perspectives in Child Care Policy.* London: Longman.

Francis, J. (1993) Elder abuse – break the silence: where do you draw the line? *Community Care,* 20 May.

Freeman, M. D. A. (1983) *The Rights and Wrongs of Children.* London: Francis Pinter.

Freeman, M. D. A. (1992) *Children, Their Families and the Law: Working with the Children Act.* London: Macmillan.

Freire, P. (1972) *Pedagogy of the Oppressed.* Harmondsworth: Penguin.

Frost, N. (1990) *Official Intervention and Child Protection: the Relationship between State and Family in Contemporary Britain.* London: Unwin Hyman.

Frost, N. (1992) Implementing the Children Act 1989 in a hostile climate, in P. Carter, T. Jeffs and M. Smith (eds), *Changing Social Work and Welfare.* Buckingham: Open University Press.

Frost, N. and Stein, M. (1989) *The Politics of Child Welfare.* Hemel Hempstead: Harvester Wheatsheaf.

Fryer, P. (1984) *Staying Power: The History of Black People in Britain.* London: Pluto Press.

Furlong, M. (1990) On being able to say what we mean: the language of hierarchy in social work practice. *British Journal of Social Work,* **20**, 575–90.

Gifford, T. (1986) *Where's the Justice?* Harmondsworth: Penguin.

Gomm, R. (1993) Issues of power in health and welfare, in J. Walmsley, J. Reynolds, P. Shakespeare and R. Woolfe (eds) *Health, Welfare and Practice: Reflecting Roles and Relationships.* London: Sage.

Griffiths, J. A. G. (1977) *The Politics of the Judiciary.* London: Fontana.

Gutierrez, L. M. (1990) Working with women of colour: an empowerment perspective. *Social Work,* March, 149–53.

Gypsy Survey (1993) *From Myth to Reality: Building Perceptions and Meeting the Need of the Gypsy Community in the 1990s.* Tyne and Wear: Northern Gypsy Council.

Halpern, A (1993) Not just a quick fix. *Community Care,* 6 May.

Hamner, J. and Statham, D. (1988) *Women and Social Work: Towards a Woman-Centred Practice.* London: Macmillan.

Hanvey, C. and Philpot, T. (1994) *Practising Social Work*. London: Routledge.

Hardiker, P., Barker, M. and Exton, K. (1989) Perspectives on prevention. *Community Care Inside*, 7 December.

Harding, T. (1993) The user speaks. *Community Care*, 11 March.

Hargrove, P. (1992) *B v B (Grandparents: Residence Order)*. *Family Law*, **22**, November, 540–1.

Harris, R. and Timms, N. (1993a) *Secure Accommodation in Child Care: Between Hospital and Prison or Thereabouts*. London: Routledge.

Harris, R. and Timms, N. (1993b). Backs against the wall. *Community Care*, 15 April, 22.

Hasenfield, Y. (1987) Power in social work practice. *Social Services Review*, **61**, 470–83.

Hayes, M. (1992) *R v Devon County Council ex parte L* [1991] 2 FLR 541 *Family Law*, **22**, June, 245–51.

Henderson, J. (1994) Reflecting oppression: symmetrical experiences of social work students and service users. *Social Work Education*, **13**(1), 16–25.

Henfrey, J. (1988) Race, in D. Hicks (ed.) *Education for Peace*. London: Routledge.

Hepinstall, D. (1992) Home truths. *Community Care*, 30 July.

Herbert, M. (1993) *Working with Children and the Children Act: a Practical Guide for the Helping Professions*. Leicester: BPS Books.

Hicks, D. (ed.) (1988) *Education for Peace*. London: Routledge.

Hill-Collins, P. (1990) *Black Feminist Thought: Knowledge, Consciousness, and the Politics of Empowerment*. London: Unwin Hyman.

HMSO (1993) *Children Act Report 1992*. London: HMSO.

Hodgson, D. (1990) *Working with the Children Act 1989. Children's Participation in Decision Making*. London: National Children's Bureau.

Holdsworth, L. (ed.) (1991) *Social Work with Physically Disabled People*. Norwich: University of East Anglia.

hooks, b. (1981) *Ain't I a Woman: Black Women and Feminism*. London: Pluto Press.

hooks, b. (1989) *Talking Back: Thinking Feminist Thinking Black*. London: Sheba.

Howe, D. (1987) *An Introduction to Social Work Theory*. London: Wildwood House.

Hughes, B. (1993) A model for the comprehensive assessment of older people and their carers. *British Journal of Social Work*, **23**, 345–64.

Jervis, M. (1989) The dilemma of intervention. *Social Work Today*, 7 December, 22.

Johnson, L. C. (1989) *Social Work Practice: a Generalist Approach*, 3rd edn. Boston: Allyn and Bacon.

Jordan, B. (1990) *Social Work in an Unjust Society*. Hemel Hempstead: Harvester Press.

Jordan, B., Karban, K., Kazi, M., Masson, H. and O'Byrne, P. (1993) Teaching values: an experience of the Diploma in Social Work. *Social Work Education*, **12**(1), 7–18.

Jordan, J. (1989) *Moving towards Home. Political Essays*. London: Virago.

Joseph, J. (1985) Warning, in *Poetry Please!* London: Everyman.

Juckes, T. J. and Barresi, J. (1993) The subjective–objective dimension in the individual–society connection: a quality perspective. *Journal for the Theory of Social Behaviour*, **23**(2), 197–216.

Kennedy, H. (1993) *Eve Was Framed. Women and British Justice*. London: Vintage Books.

Kennedy, S. (1990) Empowerment social work with physically disabled people, in L. Holdsworth (ed.) *Social Work with Physically Disabled People*. Norwich: University of East Anglia.

Kieffer, C. (1984) Citizen empowerment: a developmental perspective, in J. Rappaport, C. Swift and R. Hess (eds) *Studies in Empowerment: Steps toward Understanding and Action.* New York: Haworth Press.

King, J. (1988) Community life for ordinary people. *Community Care,* 29 September.

King, M. and Trowell, J. (1992) *Children's Welfare in the Law: the Limits of Legal Intervention.* London: Sage.

King, P. and Young, I. (1993) The child as a client. *Childright,* **95,** 15–17..

Kirton, D. and Virdee, G. (1992) *Partnership and Empowerment. Social Work with Children and Families.* Unit 12 Workbook. London: Open Polytechnic Foundation.

Kolb-Morris, J. (1993) Interacting oppressions: teaching social work content on women of colour. *Journal of Social Work Education,* **29,** 99–110.

Kopp, J. (1989) Self observation: an empowerment strategy in assessment. *Social Casework,* **60,** 276–81.

Langan, M. (1992) Introduction: women and social work in the 1990s, in M. Langan and L. Day (eds) *Women, Oppression and Social Work Issues in Anti-discriminatory Practice.* London: Routledge.

Langan, M. and Lee, P. (1989) Whatever happened to radical social work?, in M. Langan and P. Lee (eds) *Radical Social Work Today.* London: Unwin Hyman.

Lart, R. and Taylor, M. (1993) Into the melting pot. *Community Care,* 11 March.

Lee, J. A. B. (1991) Empowerment through mutual aid groups: a practice grounded conceptual framework. *Groupwork,* **4**(1), 5–21.

Leigh, J. (1992) The Child Support Act 1991: its relationship with the Children Act 1989. *Journal of Child Law,* **4**(4), 177–80.

Leonard, P. (1984) *Personality and Ideology.* London: Macmillan.

Lloyd Bostock, S. (ed.) (1979) *Psychology, Law and Legal Processes.* London: Macmillan.

Loewenstein, S. F. (1976) Integrating content on feminism and racism into the social work curriculum. *Journal of Social Work Education,* **12,** 91–6.

Lorde, A. (1984) *Sister Outsider: Essays and Speeches.* CA 95019: The Crossing Press/ Freedom.

Lowe, N. (1992) *Manchester City Council v S* (1991) 2 FLR 370. *Family Law,* **22,** January, 17–18.

Lukes, S. (1974) *Power: a Radical View.* London: Macmillan.

Lukes, S. (1986) *Power: Readings in Social and Political Theory.* Oxford: Blackwell.

Lynn, E. (1991) *Anti-Oppressive Social Work Practice Workbook.* Liverpool: John Moores University School of Law, Social Work and Social Policy.

McBarnet, D. (1981) *Conviction.* London: Macmillan.

McCluskey, J. (1993) *Reassessing Priorities. The Children Act 1989 – a New Agenda for Young Homeless People?* London: CHAR Housing Campaign for Single People.

MacDonald, S. (1991) *All Equal under the Act: a Practical Guide to the Children Act 1989 for Social Workers.* London: Race Equality Unit.

McNay, M. (1992) Social work and power relations, in M. Langan and L. Day (eds) *Women, Oppression and Social Work Issues in Anti-discriminatory Practice.* London: Routledge.

Mallinson, I. (1988) *The Social Care Task.* Social Care Association (SCA).

Marsh, P. and Fisher, M. (1992) Do we measure up? *Community Care,* 14 May.

Marchant, C. (1993) Within four walls. *Community Care,* 14 January.

Metropolitan Borough of Stockport Children's Services Division (1994/5). *Children's Services Plan.* Stockport: MBSSSD.

Mitchell, G. (1989) Empowerment and opportunity. *Social Work Today,* 16 March.

Mittler, H. (1992) Crossing frontiers. *Community Care,* 12 November.

Morgan, D. (1989) Able to intervene. *Community Care,* 30 November.

Morgan, D. and Stanley, L. (eds) (1992) *Debates in Sociology*. Manchester: Manchester University Press.

Morris, A. E. and Nott, S. N. (1991) *'Working Women and the Law': Equality and Discrimination in Theory and Practice*. London: Routledge.

Morris, J. (ed.) (1989) *Able Lives: Women's Experience of Paralysis*. London: The Women's Press.

Morris, J. (1993a) *Independent Lives? Community Care and Disabled People*. London: Macmillan.

Morris, J. (1993b) Achievable goals. *Community Care*, 18 February.

Mullender, A. and Ward, D. (1991) *Self-Directed Group Work: Users Take Action for Empowerment*. London: Whiting and Birch.

Mullender, A. and Ward, D. (1993) Empowerment and oppression: an indissoluble pairing for contemporary social work, in J. Walmsley, J. Reynolds, P. Shakespeare and R. Woolfe (eds) *Health, Welfare and Practice: Reflecting Roles and Relationships*. London: Sage.

Murray, N. (1993) Legal clout. *Community Care*, 1 July.

NACRO (1991) *The Role of Juvenile Justice Workers in Crime Prevention* (Briefing), February.

Newman, C. (1989) *Young Runaways: Findings from Britain's First Safe House*. London: The Children's Society.

Norman, A. J. (1980) *Rights and Risk*. London: Centre for Policy on Ageing.

Northern Gypsy Council (1992) Untitled collection of news items. *Northern Gypsy Voice*, Issue 1, Autumn 1992.

Norton, D. C. (1978) *The Dual Perspective*. New York: Council on Social Work Education.

Oliver, M. (ed.) (1991) *Social Work: Disabled People and Disabling Environments*. London: Jessica Kuesten Publishers.

Pahl, J. and Vaile, M. (1986) *Health and Health Care among Travellers*. Canterbury: University of Kent.

Palfrey, C., Thomas, P., Phillips, C. and Edwards, D. (1990) Jargon into practice. *Community Care*, 29 November.

Parton, N. (1985) *The Politics of Child Abuse*. London: Macmillan.

Payne, M. (1989) Open records and shared decisions with clients, in S. Shardlow (ed.) *The Values of Change in Social Work*, pp. 114–34. London: Tavistock/Routledge.

Payne, M. (1991) *Modern Social Work Theory*. London: Macmillan.

Payne, M. (1993) *Linkages: Effective Networking in Social Care*. London: Whiting and Birch.

Payne, M. (1994a) Routes to and through clienthood and their implications for practice. *Practice*, **6**(3), 169–80.

Payne, M. (1994b) The end of British social work? *Professional Social Work*, February, 5–6.

Petrie, G. (1971) *A Singular Iniquity: the Campaigns of Josephine Butler*. London: Macmillan.

Phillips, C., Palfrey, C. and Thomas, P. (1994) *Evaluating Health and Social Care*. London: Macmillan.

Phillipson, J. (1992) *Practising Equality: Women, Men and Social Work*. London: CCETSW.

Pinderhughes, E. B. (1983) Empowerment for our clients and for ourselves. *Social Casework*, **64**, 331–8.

Pitts, J. (1990) *Working with Young Offenders*. London: Macmillan.

Plummer, K. (ed.) (1992) *Modern Homosexualities*. London: Routledge.

Popay, J. and Dhooge, Y. (1989) Unemployment, cod's head soup and radical social work, in M. Langan and P. Lee (eds) *Radical Social Work Today*, pp. 140–64. London: Unwin Hyman.

Rappaport, J. (1981) In praise of paradox: a social policy of empowerment over prevention. *American Journal of Community Psychology*, **9**, 1–25.

Rappaport, J. (1984) Studies in empowerment: introduction to the issue. *Prevention in Human Services*, **3**, 1–7.

Rappaport, J. (1985) The power of empowerment language. *Social Policy*, **17**(2), 15–21.

Rappaport, J. (1987) Terms of empowerment/exemplars of prevention: toward a theory for community psychology. *American Journal of Community Psychology*, **15**(2), 121–44.

Rappaport, J., Swift, C. and Hess, R. (eds) (1984) *Studies in Empowerment: Steps toward Understanding and Action*. New York: Haworth Press.

Raths, L. E., Harman, M. and Simon, S. B. (1966) *Values and Teaching*. Columbus, OH: Charles E. Merrill.

Rees, S. (1991) *Achieving Power: Practice and Policy in Social Welfare*. Sydney: Allen and Unwin.

Rochdale Metropolitan Borough Council (1993) *Children Act under 8's Review*. Rochdale: RMBC Services and Development Plans.

Rojek, C., Peacock, G. and Collins, S. (1988) *Social Work and Received Ideas*. London: Routledge.

Rooney, B. (1987) *Racism and Resistance to Change: a Study of the Black Social Workers Project in Liverpool Social Services Department*. Liverpool: Merseyside Area Profile Group.

Rose, S. and Black, B. (1985) *Advocacy and Empowerment*. London: Routledge and Kegan Paul.

Rosenfeld, J. M. (1989) *Emergence from Extreme Poverty*. Paris: Science and Service, Fourth World Publications.

Rowe, J., Hundleby, M. and Garnett, L. (1989) *Child Care Now*. British Association of Adoption and Fostering (BAAF) Research Series 6.

Ryan, M. (1994) *The Children Act 1989: Putting It into Practice*. Hampshire: Arena Ashgate Publishing.

Sapey, B. and Hewitt, N. (1991) The changing context of social work practice, in M. Oliver (ed.) *Social Work: Disabled People and Disabling Environments*. London: Jessica Kuesten Publishers.

Seebohm Report (1968) *Report of the Committee on Local Authority and Allied Personal Social Services*. London: HMSO.

Sellick, C. (1992) *Supporting Short-term Foster Carers*. Aldershot: Avesbury.

Sennett, R. and Cobb, J. (1972) *The Hidden Injuries of Class*. New York: Vintage.

Shardlow, S. (ed) (1989) *The Values of Change in Social Work*. London: Tavistock/ Routledge.

Silcock, S. (1993) Not just a quick fix. *Community Care*, 6 May.

Simey, M. (1993) Unpublished lecture, Liverpool John Moores University.

Skidmore, R. A., Tackeray, M. G. and Farley, O. W. (1991) *Introduction to Social Work*, 5th edn. Englewood Cliffs, NJ: Prentice Hall.

Small, J. (1986) Transracial placements: conflicts and contradictions, in S. Ahmed, J. Cheetham and J. Small (eds) *Social Work with Black Children and Their Families*. London: Batsford.

Smid, G. and van Krieken, R. (1984) Notes on theory and practice in social work: a comparative view. *British Journal of Social Work*, **14**, 11–22.

Social Services Inspectorate (1992) *Court Orders Study. A Study of Local Authority Decision Making about Public Law Court Applications*. London: HMSO.

Solomon, B. B. (1976) *Black Empowerment: Social Work in Oppressed Communities*. New York: Columbia University Press.

Solomon, B. B. (1987) Empowerment: social work in oppressed communities. *Journal of Social Work Practice*, May, 79–91.

Spender, D. (1980) *Man Made Language*. London: Routledge and Kegan Paul.

Stevenson, O. and Parsloe, P. (1993). *Community Care and Empowerment*. London: Joseph Rowntree Foundation.

Stevenson, S. (1989) Taken from home, in S. Shardlow (ed.) *The Values of Change in Social Work*. London: Tavistock/Routledge.

Swift, C. (1984) Empowerment: an antidote for folly. *Prevention in Human Services*, **3**, xi–xv.

Swift, C. and Levin, G. (1987). Empowerment: an emerging mental health technology. *Journal of Primary Prevention*, **8**, 71–94.

Tatchell, P. (1992) Equal rights for all, in K. Plummer (ed.) *Modern Homosexualities*. London: Routledge.

Thompson, N. (1993) *Anti-discriminatory Practice*. London: Macmillan.

Timms, J. (1993) Forward to regional reports – practice in focus, Conference for Guardians *ad litem* and Reporting Officers.

Timms, N. (1983) *Social Work Values: an Enquiry*. London: Routledge and Kegan Paul.

Tinker, A. (1981) *The Elderly in Modern Society*, 2nd edn. London: Longman.

Tonkin, B. (1988) What the boys in the backroom will have. *Community Care*, 7 April.

Torkington, P. (1991) *Black Health: a Political Issue*. Liverpool: Catholic Association for Racial Justice and Liverpool Institute of Higher Education.

Townsend, D. (1992) New rules and new problems. *Community Care*, 26 March.

Trinder, L. (1993) For better or worse? The impact of the Children Act on court processes. *Family Law*, August 484–6.

Troyna, B. and Hatcher, R. (1992) *Racism in Children's Lives: a Study of Mainly White Primary Schools*. London: Routledge/National Children's Bureau.

Tsang, N.-M. (1993) Shifts of students' learning styles on a social work course. *Social Work Education*, **12**(1), 62–76.

Tunstil, J. (1989) Unhappy families on the sharp end. *Community Care Inside*, 7 December.

Twigg, J. and Atkin, K. (1994) *Carers Perceived*. Buckingham: Open University Press.

Ungerson, C. (1993) Caring and citizenship: a complex relationship, in J. Bornat, C. Pereira, D. Pilgrim and F. Williams (eds) *Anthology: Charter in Community Care. A Reader*, pp. 143–51. London: Macmillan/Open University.

Vernon, S. (1993) *Social Work and the Law*, 2nd edn. London: Butterworths.

Walby, C. (1993) The contract culture: mix or muddle? *Children and Society*, **7**(4), 343–56.

Walby, S. and Aaron, J. (eds) (1991) *Out of the Margins: Women Studies in the Nineties*. London: Falmer Press.

Walker, A. (1983) In search of our mothers' gardens, in P. Hill-Collins (ed.) *Black Feminist Thought: Knowledge, Consciousness and the Politics of Empowerment*. New York: Harcourt Brace Jovanovich.

Walker, A. (1991) *Recent Advances in Psychogeriatrics Volume 2*. London: Churchill Livingston.

Wallcraft, J. (1990) User involvement: how to make a success of it. *Open Mind*, 47, October/November.

Walmsley, J., Reynolds, J., Shakespeare, P. and Woolfe, R. (eds) (1993) *Health, Welfare and Practice: Reflecting Roles and Relationships*. London: Sage.

Ward, D. and Mullender, A. (1991) Empowerment and oppression: an indissoluble pairing for contemporary social work, in J. Walmsley, J. Reynolds, P.

Shakespeare and R. Woolfe (eds) *Health, Welfare and Practice: Reflecting Roles and Relationships*. London: Sage.

Ward, L. (1993) Losing out on parenthood. *Community Care*, 29 April.

Wasserstrom, R. A. (1964) Rights, human rights and racial discrimination. *Journal of Philosophy*, **61**, 628–9.

Watt, S. and Cook, J. (1993) Racism: whose liberator? Implications for women's studies, in S. Walby and J. Aaron (eds) *Out of the Margins: Women Studies in the Nineties*, pp. 131–42. London: Falmer Press.

Webb, R. and Tossell, D. (1991) *Social Issues for Carers: a Community Care Perspective*. London: Edward Arnold.

Weick, A. and Vandiver, S. (eds) (1982) *Women, Power and Change*. Washington, DC: National Association of Social Workers.

Weick, A., Rapp, C., Sullivan, W. P. and Kisthardt, W. (1989) A strengths perspective for social work practice. *Social Work*, **34**, 350–4.

Whittaker, T. (1993) Catriona Marchant. *Family Values*, 13 May, 18–19.

Wing, H. (1991) Great expectations. *Community Care Inside*, 29 August.

Yell, G. (1992) Point of order. *Law Society Gazette*, 26 August.

Zarb, G. (1991) Creating a supportive environment: meeting the needs of people who are ageing with a disability, in M. Oliver (ed.) *Social Work: Disabled People and Disabling Environments*, pp. 177–203. London: Jessica Kuesten Publishers.

INDEX

THE DEVELOPMENT OF SOCIAL WELFARE IN BRITAIN

Eric Midwinter

This textbook is aimed at undergraduate and diploma students across a wide range of the social sciences, with particular reference to those preparing for or involved in careers in social and public administration. It provides, in compact and accessible form, the story of social provision from medieval times to the present day, systematically examining major themes of:

- the relief of poverty and social care,
- healthcare and housing,
- crime and policing,
- education.

With the rise of the welfare state, and its current questioning as a chief focus, the book sets out to analyse how the state has responded to the social problems that have beset it. Consideration is given to comparative elements in Europe, North America and elsewhere, together with specific reference to issues of race, ethnicity and gender. A specially prepared glossary completes what is a well-packaged review and description of the growth and present disposition of the full range of social and public services in Britain.

Contents

Preface: How best to use this book – Introduction: Social casualty and political response – Medieval life and welfare – The nation-state and the money-economy – Industrialism's impact and the initial response – Piecemeal collectivism: Precursors of the welfare state – The silent revolution of the 1940s – The Butskellite consensus (c.1951–1973/9) – The questioning of the welfare state – General advice on further reading – Glossary of terms – Index.

208pp   0 335 19104 5 (Paperback)   0 335 19105 3 (Hardback)

IMPLEMENTING COMMUNITY CARE

Nigel Malin (ed.)

This introductory text provides a unique overview of the implementation of community care policy and the process of managing changes in the field. The central thesis is an expansion of the theme of integrating policy and professional practice in order to assess the requirements for providing models of care based upon a user and care management perspective. The book analyses the impact of changes for community nurses, social workers, those employed in residential and home-based care and discusses anticipated new roles and functions. Its examination of changes in policy and planning both at national and local level makes it a valuable sourcebook for health care, social work practitioners and planners, but the volume is designed for use by students and professionals alike. The emphasis throughout is on the design and delivery of services and providing an overview of research findings, particularly in relation to measuring service effectiveness.

Contents
Preface – Section 1: The policy context – Development of community care – Management and finance – Community care planning – Care management – Section 2: Staff and users – The caring professions – The family and informal care – Measuring service quality – The consumer role – Section 3: Models of care – Residential services – Day services – Domiciliary services – Index.

Contributors
Andy Alaszewski, Michael Beazley, John Brown, David Challis, Brian Hardy, Bob Hudson, Aileen McIntosh, Steve McNally, Nigel Malin, Jill Manthorpe, Jim Monarch, John Rose, Len Spriggs, Gerald Wistow, Wai-Ling Wun.

224pp   0 335 15738 6 (Paperback)   0 335 15739 4 (Hardback)

COMMUNITY PROFILING
AUDITING SOCIAL NEEDS

Murray Hawtin, Geraint Hughes, Janie Percy-Smith with Anne Foreman

Social auditing and community profiles are increasingly being used in relation to a number of policy areas, including: housing, community care, community health, urban regeneration and local economic development. *Community Profiling* provides a practical guide to the community profiling process which can be used by professionals involved in the planning and delivery of services, community workers, community organizations, voluntary groups and tenants' associations. In addition it will provide an invaluable step-by-step guide to social science students involved in practical research projects.

The book takes the reader through the community profiling process beginning with consideration of what a community profile is, defining aims and objectives and planning the research. It then looks at a variety of methods for collecting, storing and analysing information and ways of involving the local community. Finally it considers how to present the information and develop appropriate action-plans. The book also includes a comprehensive annotated bibliography of recent community profiles and related literature.

Contents
What is a community profile? – Planning a community profile – Involving the community – Making use of existing information – Collecting new information – Survey methods – Storing and analysing data – Collating and presenting information – Not the end – Annotated bibliography – Index.

208pp   0 335 19113 4 (Paperback)